D1292580

Power and
Illness

Power and Illness

*The Failure and Future of
American Health Policy*

Daniel M. Fox

UNIVERSITY OF CALIFORNIA PRESS
BERKELEY LOS ANGELES OXFORD

University of California Press
Berkeley and Los Angeles, California

University of California Press, Ltd.
Oxford, England

© 1993 by
The Regents of the University of California

Library of Congress Cataloging-in-Publication Data

Fox, Daniel M.
    Power and illness : the failure and future of American health
policy / Daniel M. Fox.
        p.   cm.
    Includes bibliographical references and index.
    ISBN 0-520-08409-8 (alk. paper)
    1. Medical policy—United States—History. 2. Chronically
ill—Medical care—Government policy—United States. 3. Chronic
diseases—Prevention—Government policy—United States. I. Title.
RA395.A3F685 1993
362.1'0973—dc20   93-2977
                                                               CIP

Printed in the United States of America
1 2 3 4 5 6 7 8 9

The paper used in this publication meets the minimum
requirements of American National Standard for
Information Sciences—Permanence of Paper for Printed
Library Materials, ANSI Z39.48-1984.

Contents

Acknowledgments

Many people helped me to make this book. I tested or devised most of my interpretations of past and contemporary events in conversations with colleagues. I acknowledge many of them in the Note on Methods and Sources at the end of the book. In that note, I also identify the archives and libraries where I did research in unpublished sources and to whose staffs I am grateful.

I presented most of my conclusions initially in invited lectures or articles in professional journals. Numerous listeners and reviewers asked questions and asserted alternative views that forced me to improve my understanding of events and my ability to describe them. I have credited most of the articles in the endnotes.

Gerald Grob and Rosemary Stevens, who read the book in manuscript form, made many important contributions to it. Lynne Withey has, again, been a demanding, supportive, and reliable editor.

These organizations provided financial assistance, directly or indirectly, for my research: the National Endowment for the Humanities, the Health Sciences Center of the State University of New York at Stony Brook, the Health Services Improvement Fund of Empire Blue Cross and Blue Shield, the New York State Department of Health, and the Milbank Memorial Fund. I wrote the first draft of the book during a residency at the Rockefeller Foundation's Bellagio Study Center.

During the seven years since I decided to write this book, I have had responsibility for more practical matters in health affairs. I thank John H. Marburger and J. Howard Oaks of the State University of New York at Stony Brook for tolerating my research from 1985 to 1989. Since then, my fellow directors of the Milbank Memorial Fund have encouraged me to regard this book as part of our work. I particularly appreciate the guidance of our chairman, Samuel L. Milbank. The judgments and recommendations in this book are, of course, entirely my own.

1

From Consensus to Disarray: A Century of Health Policy

The contemporary disarray in health affairs in the United States is a result of history. It is the cumulative result of inattention to the burden of chronic disabling illness. Contrary to what most people—even most experts—believe, deaths from chronic disease began to exceed deaths from acute infections almost three-quarters of a century ago. But U.S. policy, and therefore the institutions of the health sector, failed to respond adequately to that increasing burden. Today, leaders in government, business, and health affairs remain committed to policy priorities that have long been obsolete. Many of our most vexing problems in health care—soaring hospital and medical costs; limited insurance coverage, or no coverage at all, for managing chronic conditions; and the scarcity of primary care relative to specialized medical services—are the result of this failure to confront unpleasant facts.

Throughout this century, most of the people who helped make our health policy have assumed that policy should create a supply of useful scientific knowledge, specialized professionals, and facilities and equipment. On the demand side, they have assumed that policy should provide Americans with access to treatment known to prevent infectious diseases and should help them bear the costs of physician and hospital care when they are acutely ill.

During the past two decades, the persistence of this consensus—despite the changing burden of illness on the population—has contributed substantially to a policy that is largely ineffective in managing or preventing chronic illness. Changing the priorities of health policy so that resources are reallocated will require concerted, often painful, political action. Any new policy must be the result of compromises among conflicting interest groups.

These assertions summarize the story I tell in this book. I use information about the past, from the 1890s to the early 1990s, to explain the policies that Americans created to supply and pay for health services. On the basis of this analysis, I suggest more effective policies and explore the difficult politics of enacting them.

This introduction begins with a flashback to 1895 and a fast forward to 1995. Next I raise questions of method (How can historical analysis contribute to decisions about future policy?) and definition (How can the slippery phrase *chronic illness* be useful for historical and contemporary policy analysis?). Finally, I anticipate some of the recommendations about policy, and politics, that I will make in the final chapter.

Health Policy 1895

Imagine a meeting in 1895 to discuss what people a century later would describe as a policy for organizing and paying for health services. The meeting is one of a series on the same topic held in recent months in Boston, New York, Philadelphia, Baltimore, St. Louis, and Chicago. The participants are prominent physicians and leading philanthropists concerned with health and social welfare. The purpose of the meeting is to set priorities for policy in the twentieth century.[1]

The physicians are all men, mainly in their forties. Most of them have private practices, but each of them also has a faculty appointment in a medical school. A few are members or part-time employees of state or city boards of health. Almost all of them went to college for at least two years before entering medical school. After receiving their medical degrees, most of them spent a year in a laboratory or a teaching hospital in Germany, or worked under a mentor in the United States who had done so.

The philanthropists are men whose wealth is of recent origin. They made money in shipping, banking, manufacturing, and coal and petroleum extraction and refining. Although no full-time government officials, elected or appointed, attend the meeting, the philanthropists are members of boards and commissions that determine what city and state governments will spend to care for the sick and house the destitute. They also make large contributions to the campaigns of a few Democratic and more Republican candidates for public office. No women are present, though several of the men consult their female relatives before they decide about the gifts they will make in order to promote health and welfare.

There are a few clergymen in the room. Some are presidents of universities that have medical schools. Others are advisers to philanthropists.

The men quickly agree on the major problem to be addressed by health policy: preventing and alleviating the pain and poverty caused by acute infectious diseases and two chronic infections, tuberculosis and syphilis. Tuberculosis is the most threatening of these diseases, the leading cause of death and disability for most of the past century. A little more than a decade ago, in Germany, Robert Koch isolated a bacillus that most people at the meeting regard as the cause of tuberculosis. Other diseases that alarm them are diphtheria, typhoid fever, typhus, and pneumonia. There is some talk about injuries caused by the negligence of workers, and sometimes by the lax oversight of their supervisors; by the increasing numbers of vehicles on city streets; and by violence, especially in homes, streets, and saloons in the neighborhoods of recent immigrants from southern and eastern Europe.

Next they agree on the priorities of health policy. The first priority is to stimulate research in bacteriology, physiology, and related sciences. For several decades, the results of this research have increased hope that diseases caused by microbes can be prevented and cured. In France, Louis Pasteur invented a cure for rabies. Children from many countries, including the United

States, have been rushed to Paris for treatment after being bitten
by mad dogs. German investigators have recently devised an antitoxin for diphtheria. Just a year ago, during a diphtheria epidemic
in New York City, considerable quantities of this antitoxin were
distributed—for the first time anywhere—by the city's Health
Department. Only a few years before this antitoxin became available, men attending this series of meetings, the famous New York
pediatrician Abraham Jacobi for one, had watched their own
children strangle to death when the membrane that accompanies
diphtheria grew in their throats. There is no comparable treatment for tuberculosis, but this disease seems to spread less rapidly
if infected people are isolated, and if local ordinances against
public spitting reduce the amount of sputum people deposit on
sidewalks and public vehicles. Physicians attending the meeting in
New York City are winning a political battle to require their colleagues to report all persons suspected of having tuberculosis to
the Health Department, so that their sputum can be tested and
medical and social services coordinated.

The second priority is to build and renovate general hospitals
for people who are acutely ill. Unlike hospitals of the past, which
were mainly substitutes for inadequate accommodations in the
home, the modern hospital is a place where the most recent
laboratory findings are applied in the treatment of infectious disease. Decisions about admitting, diagnosing, caring for, and dis-
charging patients are now made by doctors on the basis of these
scientific findings. Lay trustees and "lady visitors" no longer believe they are entitled to participate in making these decisions, or
to make them unilaterally, as they did only a few years earlier. The
physicians at this 1895 meeting agree that the largest hospitals
should be owned or controlled by medical schools; that municipal
and voluntary hospitals should be modernized and affiliated with
these teaching institutions; and that all hospitals should be provided with the newest equipment, such as the X-ray device recently announced by Wilhelm Roentgen in Germany and reported
on enthusiastically in both the medical and the popular press.

The next priority is to reform medical schools so that they
resemble those at which the doctors who attend these meetings

hold faculty appointments. The modernized schools should emphasize the teaching of laboratory science, just as those in Germany do, and should offer supervised clinical training on the wards of teaching hospitals, as the great teaching hospitals of Britain do. The medical faculty should be appointed by universities and paid salaries for their teaching. Once appointed to a faculty, a physician should be accorded the privilege of practicing in the teaching hospital owned by or affiliated with the university. Physicians should not, as still happens at many medical schools, divide among themselves the tuition and fees that students pay. Medical schools, along with many other graduate and professional schools, should be units of the comprehensive universities being created out of older state and private institutions. Their faculties should set standards for admission and graduation and engage in scientific research as well as in teaching and patient care. The recently opened medical school and teaching hospital at the Johns Hopkins University in Baltimore is a model for others to emulate.

The men at the meeting accord the lowest priority to helping indigent people pay for medical care. Even though unemployment is still high as a result of the worldwide economic depression that began in 1893, the charity clinics and hospitals that serve the poor are raising enough money from philanthropy and city or state government to balance, if barely, their budgets. The new tuberculosis sanatoria, like the one that Edward Trudeau has established at Saranac Lake, New York, or the many that flourish in Colorado Springs, are filled with patients whose bills are paid by their families or, less often, by charitable organizations. States and cities are establishing similar sanatoria for the poor, or are creating substitutes that expose sufferers to fresh air on the roofs of hospitals or tenements. New voluntary agencies, like the visiting nurse service established in 1893 by Lillian Wald in New York, are caring for the sick poor in their own homes. The return of prosperity, expected in 1896 with the anticipated election of a Republican president to succeed Grover Cleveland, will enable most members of the middle and working classes to pay the modest out-of-pocket costs of their own health care.

In summary, the participants in the meeting agree that (in the language of the late twentieth century) the highest priorities of health policy should be to improve the supply of useful knowledge, appropriate facilities, and trained personnel. Subsidizing health care or making it affordable—that is, paying the cost of services—is not a major problem for policy.

As the men leave the meeting and pass through the corridor outside the room, they notice a display of photographs that will illustrate a pamphlet, *Health Policy 1895*, summarizing the policy recommended at the meeting. They all agree that photographs, unless deliberately distorted, are mirrors of reality. That is, they are privileged windows through which one can view past or contemporary experience. Physicians have been taking photographs and using them to illustrate lectures, textbooks, and journal articles ever since the technique for fixing images on paper was invented half a century earlier.

The men are pleased by the photographs on display, all of them recent. Most of the photographs depict surgery being performed in teaching hospitals. Modern surgery is performed in operating theaters, with each surgeon, the anesthetist, medical students, nurses, the patient, and an audience taking their appropriate roles (figure 1). No longer is most surgery performed in homes or open wards. Surgery now offers the most accessible visible imagery of modern science: surgeons, whose knowledge of anatomy and its pathology is unprecedented in history, using modern bacteriological knowledge to guard against infection.

A few photographs present care in modern hospital wards. These wards are carefully organized to implement the most advanced contemporary knowledge of infection control. Nurses, who have worn uniforms in recent decades, stand as caring guardians of the new medical order (figure 2). But physicians are really in charge in the wards, just as they are in operating theaters. When the most celebrated physician in North America, William Osler, teaches on the wards at Johns Hopkins, he is the center of attention (figure 3).

The only photograph taken outside a hospital depicts a physician reading in his modern office in a large midwestern city (figure 4). Up-to-date equipment and furniture dominate the room. No

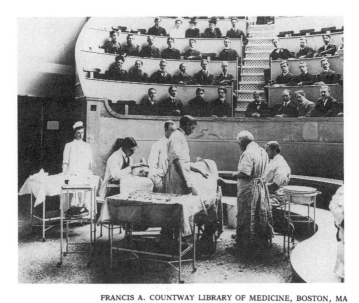

FRANCIS A. COUNTWAY LIBRARY OF MEDICINE, BOSTON, MA
Figure 1.   Amphitheater, Boston City Hospital, c. 1910

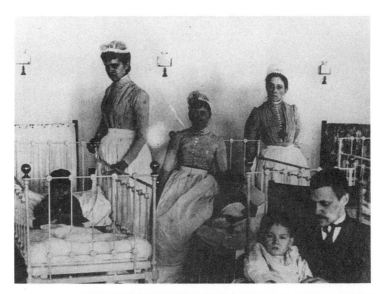

SMITHSONIAN INSTITUTION, NATIONAL MUSEUM OF AMERICAN HISTORY
Figure 2.   Pediatric ward, Bellevue Hospital, New York, 1900

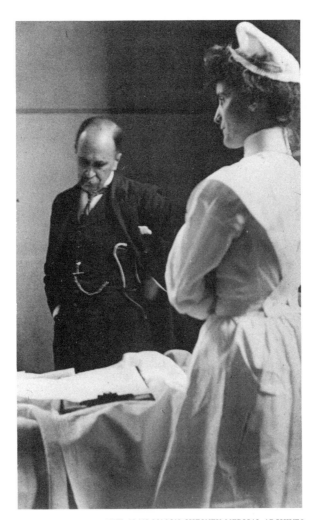

THE ALAN MASON CHESNEY MEDICAL ARCHIVES
OF THE JOHNS HOPKINS MEDICAL INSTITUTIONS

Figure 3.   Medical ward, Johns Hopkins Hospital, Baltimore, c. 1895

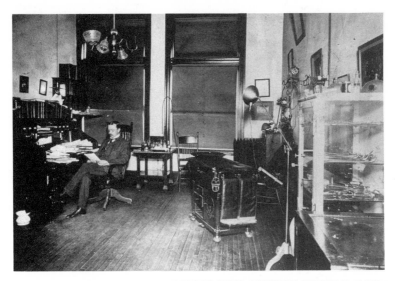

THE FLASHLIGHTERS PHOTO, MINNESOTA HISTORICAL SOCIETY

Figure 4.   Physician's office, Minneapolis, c. 1900

patient is present. Physicians and their patients are photographed together only in small-town offices or in hospital wards for low-income patients. Urban physicians and their affluent patients regard medical encounters as separate from ordinary life; photographs resembling those taken on social occasions make them uncomfortable.

The photographs on the wall, taken together, offer a coherent visualization of the priorities of health policy. The participants routinely look at other contemporary photographs about health care. They see many pictures of, for example, persons with tuberculosis being cared for in sanatoria or, if they are poor, seeking fresh air on the roofs of tenements or hospitals. They are familiar with photographs of nurses visiting bedridden patients in the slums. But they do not regard these as *medical* pictures that should be displayed and published to support recommendations for policy. Such images are best used to illustrate the fund-raising brochures of charities that assist poor people for whose diseases medicine still must find explanations and treatments. The photographs that will illustrate the pamphlet confirm the policy agreements reached at the recent meeting.

Health Policy 1995

Now imagine a meeting about the priorities of health policy in 1995. Many more people are in a much larger room, in Washington, D.C. They include representatives of about seventy medical specialty and subspecialty societies and about a hundred other licensed professions, the largest of which is nursing. A group of Ph.D.s attend on behalf of physiology, cellular and molecular biology, biochemistry, and the other basic medical sciences. Many service providers also are present: managers of large hospitals and their affiliated health care systems and of health maintenance organizations, nursing homes, and home health care agencies; representatives of corporations that make and sell pharmaceuticals, medical supplies, and equipment; and members of the trade associations created by each of these groups. Instead of the large contingent of philanthropists who attended the earlier meeting, a few foundation presidents attend as observers. Almost all of them are physicians or social scientists. Other observers include a few economists and ethicists, most of whom work at universities or private research organizations.[2]

Representatives of another group, people who purchase and pay for health services, were not present at the meeting in 1895. These people include officials of federal, state, and local government; nonprofit and commercial insurance companies; and some of the largest corporations in the country, which "self-insure" to pay for their employees' health care. These purchasers of care are accompanied by representatives of firms that assist them in making and controlling payment—people, for example, who process data, pay bills, collect premiums, and authorize or review the use of services.

A few people introduce themselves as representatives of consumers. Some of them speak on behalf of people with particular diseases or disabling conditions. Others claim to represent minority groups, women, children, the elderly, or what they call the "public interest." Still others represent unions, mainly of public employees, service industry employees, and automobile workers.

Many lawyers are present. Some work for people who call

themselves providers, others for payers. Off to one side, talking only with members of their own group, are trial lawyers who specialize in malpractice claims.

Hundreds of print and electronic journalists attend the meeting. Most of them regularly cover health and medical affairs, either for the general press and television or for large-circulation weeklies published by professional and trade associations in health affairs. Each of the speakers begins and ends with a brisk thirty-second summary, during which he or she glances at the press table to see who is taking notes and which cameras are in play.

The participants in the meeting agree about the priorities for health policy; but they disagree, often strongly, about the relative importance of these priorities. The leaders of each group of providers and payers make coherent, informed, and passionate arguments. The words *access*, *quality*, and *cost* are repeated many times. Every time the participants seem to reach consensus that health policy should emphasize research, hospitals, and primary and long-term care, somebody precipitates renewed controversy by talking about the importance of controlling costs. Then a debate ensues about the relative effectiveness of different ways to cut costs: setting global budgets, regulating physicians' and hospitals' prices, reducing administrative costs, and applying the results of research on the outcomes of alternative treatments.

There is, however, considerable agreement about the underlying problems that drive health policy. People are living longer and as a result are suffering more chronic disabling illnesses, which require both continuous management and intervention in acute episodes. Some people remember that, for two decades before the recognition of AIDS in 1981, many experts, even a surgeon general of the United States, said that we knew how to solve the problems of infectious disease. Now it is clear that AIDS itself is a disease of long duration and considerable cost and must be regarded as a chronic infectious disease. It is like tuberculosis except that it remains uncurable.

The participants have conflicting opinions about the health policy reforms of the Clinton administration and the half-dozen or so state initiatives that preceded them. Everyone is pleased that more people are now insured for basic physician and hospital services. But others complain that access to acute care is still not universal and that long-term care is being ignored. Others predict that current cost-containment policy will not be strong enough. Still others assert that the policy restricts freedom of choice by physicians and patients and is stifling innovation in treatment. Similarly, some participants applaud the new incentives for physicians to enter primary care practice; but others believe that these measures, along with cost ceilings, will inevitably lead to rationing, which the public will find intolerable.

The meeting ends in polite disarray. The participants have met before and will meet again in what seems an interminable quest for consensus and the achievement of each group's goals. Unlike the participants at the 1895 meeting, everyone at this meeting places her or his own bet on the future, and then promptly places another as a hedge.

As in 1895, photographs are displayed in the corridor outside the meeting room. These photographs will not, however, be published with the proceedings of the meeting. Just as the participants could not agree on the hierarchy of priorities for policy, they are divided about an appropriate imagery for contemporary health care. The photographs were in fact chosen to represent the diversity of contemporary images of health care. They were selected by a curator from the International Center for Photography in New York City, who intended to display both diversity and the high aesthetic standards of contemporary documentary photography. A label alongside each picture names the photographer who took it. In 1895, the photographers were anonymous; their names did not matter, since they took pictures where and when physicians told them to. In 1995, in contrast, the photographers and the agencies representing them have control over the images they make and where and how they are displayed.

Each of the images is unsettling; each, that is, seems to raise questions about the adequacy of contemporary health policy. William Strode's photograph of a patient having a liver scan, for instance, might communicate uncertainty about whether the

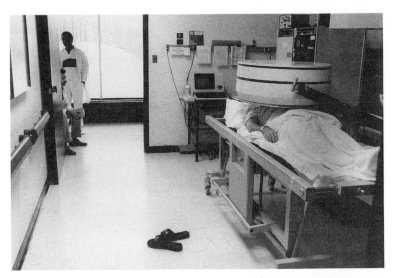

WILLIAM STRODE/WILLIAM STRODE ASSOCIATES
Figure 5.   Liver scan, University Hospital, Stony Brook, New York

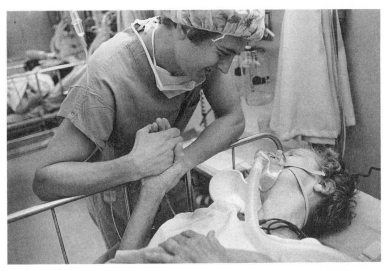

EUGENE RICHARDS/MAGNUM
Figure 6.   Hospital, Boston, from Dorothea Lynch and Eugene Richards, *Exploding into Life* (New York: Aperture, 1986)

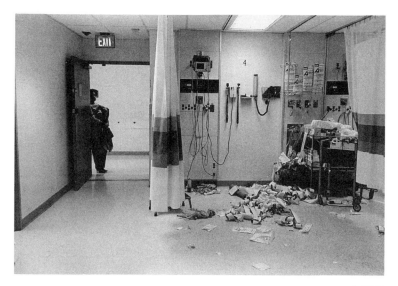

SYLVIA PLACHY © 1993
Figure 7.   After a heart attack, Booth Memorial Hospital, New York

expensive procedure will yield signs of disease and whether effective treatment is possible (figure 5). The patient in intensive care
in Eugene Richards's photograph (figure 6) is dying; what does
the surgeon's personal warmth accomplish?

Two other photographs are more explicitly critical of health
policy. Sylvia Plachy's emergency surgical suite suggests the futility and exhaustion of technological competence (figure 7). Mel
Rosenthal, juxtaposing a homeless man and the entrance to a
hospital emergency room, questions the appropriateness of contemporary resource allocation (figure 8).

The events at this meeting are communicated to a larger audience than the physicians and philanthropists who received the
pamphlet published in 1895. A videotape of highlights is televised
later that week on the Public Broadcasting System, with guest
commentary by a news anchorperson from a commercial network. Editorials about it appear in the *New York Times*, the
Washington Post, and other leading newspapers. On television
and in the press, commentators agree that health policy must be

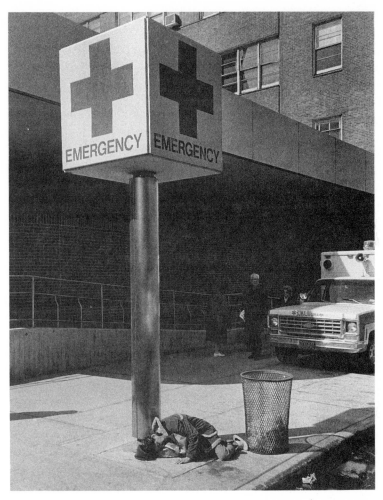

MEL ROSENTHAL/TRIAGE PROJECT

Figure 8. Hospital emergency entrance, New York

reformed and that firm leadership will be required in negotiations among contending parties. A few weeks later, a leading opinion-polling firm reports that the American people regard improved access to health care as an important issue; but, the pollsters report, health is still not as important to most Americans as jobs, income, taxes, and peace.

History Matters: The Methods of This Book

Most of the participants in the imaginary meeting of 1995 would not know or care that, a century earlier, there had been consensus about the priorities of health policy. It has become unfashionable to regard history as an important source of practical knowledge for people who make policy or even for those who study it. Because they do not know that there was consensus in the past, the 1995 participants have no interest in knowing why and how this consensus was created and sustained, how it eventually disintegrated, or what this history might tell them about possible alternatives for contemporary policy.

In this book, I try to persuade readers that history matters for making decisions about policy in the present and the future. Most of my professional colleagues are people who help to make health policy or who write about it. Many of them, even people for whom I have admiration and even affection, are prisoners of an unexamined past. For these colleagues, the past is what they and their professional and political allies remember: the anecdotes and generalizations that are called, in contemporary jargon, "institutional memory," or, less pompously, "war stories." For others, the past is boring and irrelevant; since elementary school, they have been convinced that history is just "one damn thing after another."

The history that people remember is almost always self-serving. It consists of stories—about events or professions or interest groups—that serve the purposes of those who tell and listen to the stories. These purposes are usually harmless: people remembering the old days, often with nostalgia; older men and women reminding young colleagues that giants once walked the earth. But sometimes remembered history is pernicious. It prevents storytellers and their listeners from understanding the full complexity of what happened, why it happened, and with what effects. Remembered history can absolve people from accountability for actions based on precedents that have lost their relevance for the present—so that, for example, medical students' clinical experience consists almost entirely of work with patients who have acute conditions and are seen in hospitals or their adjacent clinics. This practice made sense in 1895, when physicians in offices and dispensaries provided a great deal of unscientific acute care. But it persists a century later, supported by state appropriations for higher education and endorsed by a national accrediting agency. Now, however, most physicians use the knowledge they acquired in medical schools and teaching hospitals to help their patients manage chronic conditions in community settings.

Here are two more examples of how remembered history can impede critical analysis. Many people believe that, at least since the birth of modern biological science, physicians have always been better paid and more respected than members of other professions. These people are unlikely to ask how and why physicians became wealthy and powerful and whether their continued ascendancy is essential in order to have an effective system of health care.[3] Similarly, many people remember that for most of the twentieth century the purpose of laboratory research in medical science has been to expand basic knowledge. They see no need to inquire whether public expenditures for research have had any relationship to the inadequacy of practical knowledge about the course of chronic disease.[4] Assumptions based on historical memory alone are usually false.

The remedy for the failures of remembered history is analytical history, the method known as "historical science" in other languages than English. Professional historical study, like work in most other scientific disciplines, is conducted mainly for its own sake. Most professional scholars or scientists are properly suspicious of becoming propagandists or apologists. In addition, professional historians have a particular concern about what they call "presentism"—that is, distorting the study of the past by retroactively asking questions derived from current events.

Even though most scientific inquiry, in every discipline, is conducted for its own sake, it is always shadowed by ideology and opinion. According to a great deal of scholarship in the history and sociology of science, researchers have not been able to liberate themselves from normative models of the goals of science and, often, of society. Peer review can reduce but not eliminate subjectivity.[5]

A scholar or scientist who tries to use knowledge to inform policy often evokes skepticism among his or her colleagues. Many historians and other social scientists, as well as people in other fields, have become defenders of the status quo or advocates of revolutions against it. There are no neat solutions to the problems of using science and scholarship for public purposes.[6]

Nor are there any simple remedies for the selective perception of evidence. The best remedy I have found is to state my bias. It is as follows: I believe that members of a society share moral and financial responsibility for alleviating pain and suffering. I also believe that the leaders of every institution, whether nominally in the private or the nonprofit or the public sector, must always consider the broad public interest. But I am agnostic about how government and markets, separately or in combination, should be used to solve particular individual and social problems. I also believe, of course, that clear, honest thinking and good information can be useful for solving these problems.

Consensus and Conflict in the History of Health Policy

Continuity and changes in health policy are caused by ideas, interests, and illness, in complex interaction. Most people who have explained the history and politics of health policy have given priority first to ideas, then to interests, and then to the two in reciprocal relationship. Few have examined the effect of illness on policy, either alone or in combination with ideas and interests. One of the few who has is Rosemary Stevens, who writes, for example, that "complex health (and public health) problems will remain largely unexamined while incurable diseases . . . remain on the fringes of medical prestige."[7]

I came only gradually to understand the importance of studying the relationship among ideas, interests, and illness. In 1986, in a book titled *Health Policies, Health Politics: The Experience of Britain and America,* I described the importance of ideas in shaping the interests that groups brought to negotiations about health policy. This interpretation contradicted two generalizations that had dominated scholarship in the field for a generation: (1) that conflicts among interest groups composed mainly of providers and consumers of care determined how health services were organized and financed; (2) that the ideas most relevant in making health policy had to do with equity, collective responsibility, social efficiency, and conflicts among social classes. These ideas had been the basis for the creation of welfare state policies in Europe and, in a much weaker way, in the United States.[8]

I devised alternative interpretations. I claimed that consensus was more important than conflict in making health policy in the twentieth century because of different ideas. The ideas that mattered most were technological assumptions about medicine rather than principles of general welfare. That is, the most influential ideas were about achieving better health for individuals and populations as a result of applying the methods and findings of laboratory and clinical science. Health policy and politics, I concluded, had been privileged, set apart as a special area of public concern. Health policy, people assumed, held so much promise for human progress that the most important decisions about it could be made by physicians, with minimal oversight by outsiders.

Then I realized that I had ignored a major issue. I had written about ideas and interests as if changes in the illnesses that made people sick and disabled and eventually killed them did not matter very much for policy. I began to recognize this error when I read that, according to the United States Census, most recorded deaths in 1920 had been caused by chronic degenerative diseases, notably cancer, diabetes, kidney disease, and lung disease (not heart disease, which was then regarded as mainly infectious in origin).[9] I had failed to understand that the assumptions governing health policy in the United States and Western Europe in the twentieth century were beginning to be obsolete by 1920. They were becoming obsolete even before they had been translated into policy and thus into unprecedented expenditures for health services by government and philanthropy. But for more than half a century after 1920, health policy was made as if its central problem still was and would remain the conquest of infectious disease and the acute episodes that were common to both raging infections and particular, usually advanced, stages of chronic illness. Institutions that were shaped by policy to give priority to this misstated problem included hospitals, research laboratories, medical schools, and health insurance plans. These institutions would, however, increasingly spend their resources, often grudgingly, to resolve different problems: managing the long course of the chronic illnesses with which most of their patients presented themselves. The institutions would accommodate to patients with chronic illness mainly by taking care of them when their afflictions most closely resembled infections; that is, in their acute episodes and end stages. Patient education, rehabilitation, and the accommodation of homes and workplaces to the functional limitations of persons with disabling conditions received lower priority.

This was a new way to interpret the history of health services and policy: leaders in health affairs had avoided taking account of evidence about changing characteristics of the burden of illness. Why did they avoid this pressing issue? How did policy eventually take account of the results of changes in the burden of illness? After reading many archival and published primary sources, I decided that two big stories about twentieth-century health policy must be told. One story was about the gradual accommodation of professions, institutions (especially hospitals), and payment systems to the inexorable increase in death and disability from chronic illness and injury. The other story was about the persistence of policy priorities elaborated between the 1890s and the 1920s and the power of the interest groups that found satisfaction, prestige, and wealth in acting on those priorities.

Slippery Words

In the preceding discussion of methods and models, I have used a number of words and phrases that require more precise definition. I begin with simpler terms and proceed, in the next section, to my major task: establishing a definition of chronic illness that is both consistent with human experience and useful for the analysis in this book.

By *health policy*, one of the organizing phrases for this book, I mean deliberate efforts to prevent, postpone, treat, or accommodate to illness or injury for significant groups of people, usually within firms or political jurisdictions. Health policy is made and implemented by persons who are employed by public and private organizations; the latter include commercial enterprises and voluntary, nonprofit associations. For convenience, I divide policies, using a construct borrowed from economics, into those that affect the supply of health services (such as research, education, and the construction of hospitals and other facilities) and those that affect the demand for care (for instance, coverage by voluntary and social insurance, or out-of-pocket costs).

My use of the words *ideas, interests,* and *illness* is a device for communicating with diverse audiences. By *ideas,* I mean values, ideologies, and operating assumptions. Values are strongly held opinions about the purposes of human beings and societies. Ideologies—or, more accurately, political principles—are criteria for interpreting events and acting to shape them; people derive these criteria from their values. Operating assumptions are untestable opinions, based on values and ideologies, about how the world works. These assumptions include opinions about the significance of science and technology or of such socioeconomic arrangements as classes, races, ethnic groups, markets, corporations, or nonprofit associations.

The word *interests* is much easier to define. I use it to mean what individuals, usually acting through associations, unions, or political parties, believe to be good for themselves.

Illnesses are the events—some well understood, others less so—that cause impairment, disability, and death in individuals and, in the aggregate, in populations. The words *acute, chronic, illness, disability,* and *disease* have imprecise and often overlapping definitions. *Acute* has usually described particularly painful experiences of infection or injury and the consequences of chronic degenerative biological processes. The phrases *chronic illness* and *chronic disease* are often used interchangeably. *Disability* usually refers to an inability to work or to engage in other activities of daily life as a result of a chronic impairment that resulted from disease, injury, or genetic anomalies; but it has frequently been used as a synonym for chronic disease.[10]

These definitions are inexact because disease and disability are not precise entities that can be defined entirely by their biological characteristics. People make diseases and disabilities by defining biological phenomena, individual reactions to them, and social or environmental conditions in particular ways at different times.

The Meanings of Chronic Illness

The concept of chronic disease (or chronic illness) has both an ancient and a modern history. Since antiquity, physicians and their patients have recognized that some afflictions appear suddenly and rage briefly, leaving their victims weak, disfigured, or dead. They also observed that other afflictions have a slow onset and lead to increasing disability and, frequently, death. For several thousand years, plague and various fevers exemplified the first category; cancer and insanity, the second.

The modern history of chronic illness began during the eighteenth and nineteenth centuries. Two sets of events are central to this history. The first was the changing pattern of disease in Europe and North America. The second was the changing understanding of the causes and course of disease (and the use of the word *disease* itself with greater precision) as a result of advances in biological and chemical knowledge. The two sets of events merged in the late nineteenth century to create an optimistic consensus about the future of health policy.

In retrospect, it is now evident that in the eighteenth century people in Europe and North America began, in historian Ann

Carmichael's useful phrase, to "distance their exposure" to both acute (e.g., plague) and chronic (e.g., tuberculosis) infectious disease.[11] According to historians, the number of deaths directly attributable to infection gradually declined because of better access to food; public health intervention to clean the environment; and changes in personal behavior, including more frequent bathing and handwashing and the covering of one's mouth and nose when sneezing. This gradual decline in the burden of infections went unnoticed by most contemporaries, especially since in Western Europe urban mortality from infections increased as a result of economic dislocations that accompanied industrialization in the first half of the nineteenth century.

In the second half of that century, the growing perception that the threat of infection was receding coincided with the ascendancy of new theories for understanding disease and intervening to prevent and treat it. Most important, the great advances in bacteriology in these years led to the concept, in the words of a classic study of human disease, that "each human ailment must have a singular and specific cause."[12] For the next century, medical scientists regularly announced the singular, specific bacterium, environmental toxin, or virus that was implicated in a specific disease. Most of the diseases for which singular, specific causes were announced seemed only to have acute phases. Individuals experienced some of these diseases (such as diphtheria or cholera) only once; others (such as malaria) could be experienced recurrently. The great exceptions were the major chronic infectious diseases, tuberculosis and syphilis.

The phrase *chronic disease* soon came to be used by most physicians, however, mainly as a loose descriptor for illnesses of slow onset and long course, for which a singular and specific cause had not yet been discovered. This usage was well established in medical and popular publications by the end of the nineteenth century. For example, *chronic disease* became a standard label for the underlying, if poorly understood, causes of most people's deaths. In this usage, a chronic ailment was said to have weakened the patient; an acute illness then caused his or her death. A related usage persists at present, when chronic disease is often the primary cause of death. For instance, the editor of a massive reference book published in 1993, *The Cambridge World History of Human Disease*, wrote that "in the developed world, chronic diseases . . . have supplanted infectious diseases as the important killers, and increasingly the role of genes in the production of these diseases has come under scrutiny."[13] There is no further discussion of chronic disease in general in the book, though many of its authors routinely use the phrase as I do here.

The inescapable imprecision of language that describes disease creates several problems for me and for readers of this book. The most important of these problems is whether my central distinction, between chronic and acute illness, is merely a matter of shifting definitions, and not a major issue for policy. The distinction is, I believe, quite real. Throughout the past century, statisticians, epidemiologists, physicians, and most policy makers have used the distinction between chronic and acute illness with reasonable precision. They have written and acted with considerable agreement about the characteristics of a category of diseases they called "chronic" because of the way they affect people. These diseases gradually impair the functions of organs and cause disability that can be described accurately as either progressive, in remission, or causing "acute" distress. The underlying causes of these chronic diseases include bacteria, viruses, genes, environmental toxins, injuries, and the unexplained degeneration of organs and organ systems, often as a result of the biology of aging.

A second problem for this book is whether the burden of chronic illness has in fact been changing during the past century. The commonsense answer, "Of course it has," will not quite do. Certainly there were changes in the reported incidence and prevalence of chronic disease relative to acute infectious disease. Of course, changes in what is reported do not necessarily constitute changes in what has occurred. There is, however, convincing evidence that, on a population basis, both actual and reported cases of many acute infectious diseases have declined; that the prevalence of particular chronic diseases has increased as more people live longer; and that the incidence of many chronic diseases—lung cancer, for instance—has increased.

The final problem concerns the inclusion of mental illness, the chronic affliction for which there is the longest history of provision in public policy. For expediency, I discuss mental illness only when its burden raises issues about general policy for supplying and meeting the demand for health services. For example: Should treatment of mental illness be covered by insurance? When does policy for research on mental illness become part of general health research policy? How do ideas about policy for mental illness influence the course of policy for other chronic diseases? This expedient decision was mainly arbitrary. I made it to avoid adding further bulk to an already dense book. The decision also reflects the relative segregation of policy and treatment for mental illness from general health policy during most of the past century. My decision was, however, made considerably easier because many good studies—especially a recent book by Gerald Grob[14]—are available on the history of policy for mental illness.

In sum, this book has at its core a somewhat ambiguous but nevertheless useful concept, chronic illness. Like all illnesses, those that are chronic have causes and consequences that are both biological and social.

So What? And Other Practical Questions

If I have persuaded some readers that this book has a significant subject and others that historical social science has merit, I may still have alienated prospective readers who matter very much to me. These are people who lack the time or the patience to read books about health issues that do not have practical conse-quences. I have, however, written this book mainly because I spend my professional life working to improve health policy in the United States. The question that dominates the book is "What about the future?" Robert J. Maxwell, a businessman and social scientist who is also chief executive officer of a major British philanthropic foundation, asked this question in a review of my book comparing the history of health policy in the United States and the United Kingdom. Maxwell went on to say that "Fox disarmingly refuses to pass any judgment or to make any predictions." How, he asked, should we make "hard choices" about health policy, choices that are "economic, scientific, behavioral, political and ethical"?[15]

In this book, I pass judgment and venture predictions. I assert that for three-quarters of a century interest groups in health affairs have responded, often reluctantly, to the increasing incidence and prevalence of chronic disabling illness. But this response, I believe, has been inadequate and has not transformed the priorities of health policy. Instead, support continues to be strong for priorities set a century ago. These priorities translate into two leading goals for health services: prolonging life and alleviating pain. Much health policy, especially for financing health services, accords these goals higher priority than preventing or postponing disease, disability, and premature death. The general acceptance of these outmoded priorities is evidenced in the frequent debates, well reported in the media, about whether expensive medical care should be rationed. The participants in these debates usually argue about whether we can afford to give expensive health care to all people, whatever their age and physical or mental capacity. The issues and stakes are familiar, especially the difficulties of deciding whether and how to ration access to expensive medical technology for people whose illnesses are terminal.

A more important practical question, however, for a society struggling to adapt to its burden of chronic disabling illness is how to enable the largest possible number of people to live independently and productively. Most people are mainly concerned about preventing disease and disability and getting assistance for the illnesses and injuries they suffer. Addressing these issues adequately will require an exceedingly difficult redistribution of the resources currently spent for health services.[16]

There are two practical reasons to emphasize policy for *how* people live rather than *who* shall live. The first reason is that many, perhaps most, decision makers, whether they are physicians, or insurers or public officials, find it repugnant to make policies that do not prolong life whenever possible or that wrench decisions about life and death away from patients and their families in consultation with their physicians. As a result, the debate, however stirring, is in practice sterile. The second reason is that decisions about whether to use heroic measures and expensive technologies for particular individuals are most often the cumulative result of years of neglecting the prevention, postponement, and management of chronic illness.

Before anticipating the recommendations that I will make at the end of this book to enhance the political feasibility of redistributing resources for health care, I want to deny any intent to bash the medical profession. I know from much experience as a speaker and writer that I am likely to be misunderstood on this point. In actuality, however, I strongly endorse both the continuing prominence of physicians in personal health services and the high priority given to medical research. Advocacy by clinicians, medical scientists, and epidemiologists has been responsible for much of the attention to chronic illness in health policy since the 1920s. As I describe in the next chapter, people in these fields understood the significance of chronic disabling illness for policy long before most of their colleagues in public health and hospital administration, health insurance, and even many specialties of medicine did.

My recommendations for new policy assume that the issues in health affairs that currently occupy most of our attention will be resolved, and that we can then consider more difficult issues. I am betting, that is, that sometime in the 1990s, after much debate and negotiation, the United States will enact health policies that will enable almost everyone to have access to basic medical and hospital services. These policies will almost surely include elements from a number of competing schemes put forth by reformers. There will, for example, be competition among payers and providers, but it will be managed. Health insurance will probably remain linked to employment, but risks will be pooled in ways that reduce the vulnerability of sick people who work in small firms or who have low incomes. Some of the reforms will be national, others will be made within the states, and still others will be made by private employers. Like any political compromise, the new policy for access will leave many groups unsatisfied.

Then, for the first time, we will be able to make and implement
coherent policies for preventing and managing chronic illness. As
a result of these reforms in access to care, almost all U.S. citizens
will probably be enrolled in a health plan of sufficient size to bear
the high costs of their catastrophically expensive and severely
disabling illnesses and injuries. The next problems for policy will
be to reduce the incidence and prevalence of these catastrophes
by prevention, treatment, and rehabilitation. This reduction will
be limited by what turn out to be realistic expectations for mortality.

Solving these problems will be expensive. The best way to cover
the expenses is to redistribute resources within the health sector.
There are two inviting, but well-protected, targets for initial redistribution: excess capacity in acute general hospitals and a perverse
ratio of subspecialized to primary care physicians. The politics of
redistribution will be nasty. But redistribution may, in the end, be
less damaging than increasing the percentage of national product
that we spend for health care at the expense of education, infra-
structure, housing, and, perhaps most important, economic
growth.

During the past decade, many decision makers, especially private employers, were surprised to discover that spending for
health services had been increasing rapidly for a generation. There
was no good reason for them to be surprised. Health has become
as pressing a public concern as national security and the economy.
Health services are expensive largely because of the incidence and
prevalence of chronic disabling illness and the general willingness
in this country to do something about it, especially in its acute
stages. To a large extent, but not entirely, the growing burden of
chronic illness is a result of an aging population. The growth of the
health sector is only in a limited, if still very expensive, way a
result of the greed and power of interest groups that took advantage of generous reimbursement under voluntary and social insurance and large public subsidies.

In the future, leaders of the executive and legislative branches
of government and of the private sector are likely to give more
attention to health policy than they did over the past century.

Most of the attention accorded to health policy by leaders of general government and the economy, especially in the past generation, has been the result of crises. Memorable crises have occurred over the access of the elderly, the poor, and the uninsured to affordable services; or over epidemics of influenza, polio, and AIDS; or over budget shortfalls in cities and states. Crises will continue to occur, but they may be less important than the perception that health policy is important for maintaining and enhancing productivity as well as civic and family life. These concerns are too important to our society to leave them to experts, professionals, and interest groups, as we have for most of the past century.

Solving problems of this magnitude will require changes in familiar patterns of authority and accountability in the health sector. These patterns persist as a result of the historical events I now describe. Changing them will result in new priorities and policies and new ways of thinking about what we have up to now separated as public health and personal health services.

2

The Paradox of Health
Policy, 1900-1950

For most of the twentieth century, the United States has spent private and public funds generously in order to increase the supply and availability of health care. But this generosity has not been accurately directed at the needs of the American people, as revealed by the causes of their sickness and death. That is the paradox of health policy.

In the mid-twentieth century, most Americans grew increasingly confident about their prospects for improved health. But their optimism was misplaced. They were living longer, but not necessarily healthier, lives. In the decade after World War II, the priorities of health policy and Americans' experience of illness in fact diverged more widely than at any other time in this century. Health policy accorded priority to expanding access to acute care. Consequently, more people were now covered by voluntary health insurance, and general hospitals proliferated. Moreover, additional subsidies were provided for research and the training of specialist physicians. At the same time, the incidence and prevalence of chronic illness and disability, which had been increasing for a generation, accelerated.

At the turn of the century, in contrast (as noted in chapter 1), the experience of disease was congruent with the priorities of policy. Acute infectious diseases were the leading causes of sickness and death. Preventing and curing them properly had priority in health policy. Following the advice of academic physicians, policy makers—mainly philanthropists and officials of state and local government—supported research; increased public health work in surveillance, prevention, and treatment; and, most important, subsidized a rapid increase in the availability of hospital services and specialized medical care—all in the interest of fighting acute infectious disease. Although, as the century progressed, Americans had increasing cause for concern about sickness, disability, and death from chronic degenerative diseases—notably cancers, heart disease, stroke, and diabetes—health policy continued to give priority to research and public health programs that targeted infections and to hospital and medical services for acute, life-threatening episodes of infectious and degenerative disease.

Most of the people who made and influenced policy assumed that the institutions and methods that seemed to be succeeding against acute infectious disease could be effective in the struggle against death and disability from chronic degenerative conditions. The discovery of insulin treatment for diabetes in the 1920s seemed to prove the effectiveness of existing methods and priorities in medical research. So did the announcement in 1949 that a cortical steroid, with the trade name Cortisone, caused prompt remission of the symptoms of rheumatoid arthritis, the most prevalent chronic disease. These breakthroughs convinced many people of the effectiveness of policies that established hierarchies of laboratories, teaching hospitals, specialized medical practices, community hospitals, and general medical care.

Since the 1920s, however, a number of people who were prominent in health affairs had advocated higher priority to chronic illness. These people were medical scientists and statisticians, practicing physicians and public health officers. They urged new policies for research, prevention, and the management of patients through the long course of their disabling illnesses. In the 1930s, as a result of their efforts, the institutions of the health sector began gradually to accommodate to the new epidemiological situation.

The contemporary experience of illness could not, however, be addressed adequately without fundamental changes in policy for financing personal health services. Chronic illness placed heavy financial burdens on individuals and families and, for people who were poor or were pauperized by illness, on philanthropy and government. These costs could be predicted by actuaries using epidemiological data. The costs could be made bearable for individuals and families if they were distributed among large groups of people through insurance premiums, charity, and public appropriations. But the politics of health care in the United States made it difficult both to create risk pools that were sufficiently large and diverse to meet the costs of treating chronic illness and to provide charity or public subsidy for people who could not afford private insurance.

By 1950, in sum, the powerful ideas and interests that would shape health policy in the second half of the century were securely established. Both the ideas and the interests were, however, inadequate to address the increasing burden of chronic illness.

Changes in Causes of Death and Disability

A rapid and unexpected change in the leading causes of death and disability occurred early in the twentieth century. In 1914, the Committee on Public Health of the New York Academy of Medicine reported that "more people die from chronic disease than from acute." Moreover, the "proportion would undoubtedly be much higher than the mortality statistics indicate if every death certificate . . . showed the chronic disease which is largely responsible for the fatal result."[1] Even though contemporary mortality statistics were not entirely accurate, they revealed unanticipated changes in the burden of illness. In 1900, the leading causes of death were "pneumonia and influenza, tuberculosis, [and] diarrhea, enteritis and ulceration of the intestines."[2] The participants in the imaginary summit meeting of 1895 described in chapter 1 would have been pleased though hardly surprised by this additional evidence of the appropriateness of their priorities for health policy.

Forty years later, however, in 1940, the three leading causes of death were chronic degenerative conditions: "diseases of the heart, cancer and other malignant tumors, [and] intracranial lesions of vascular origin."[3] Sixty years later, in 1960, only nomenclature had changed. The three leading causes of death were now "diseases of the heart, malignant neoplasms, [and] vascular lesions affecting [the] central nervous system."[4] These would remain among the leading causes of death for the rest of the century.

To compare causes of illness and death over time, a colleague and I aggregated statistics from the United States during the first half of the century.[5] Beginning with the more accessible data in the census using the crude death-rate figures, we found that, in 1900, 24.4 percent of total deaths could be attributed to chronic diseases. By 1940, the rate had increased to 61.2 percent. We then employed a statistical technique to take account of the possibility that the increased mortality from chronic disease had occurred because more people were surviving their childhood illnesses and living into old age. In 1900, 28.1 percent of the age-adjusted death rate was attributable to chronic diseases; by 1940, that figure had risen to 56.9 percent. We continued this table until 1948, when the rate was 64 percent. Revised international conventions for coding diseases prevented us from comparing causes of death after 1948 with those that occurred earlier in the century. The imprecisely comparable data for 1960, however, showed 57.7 percent of deaths occurring as a result of chronic disease.

The pain and deprivation of everyday life are captured better by information about illness (technically, about morbidity and disability) than by data about the causes of death. But data about morbidity and disability before the 1950s are limited in amount and difficult to compare. Most of the morbidity statistics from the nineteenth century describe claims requesting payment by insurance funds for lost wages, rather than the morbidity and disability that individuals experienced.[6] Similarly, the extensive morbidity studies conducted in the first four decades of the twentieth century—notably by the Metropolitan Life Insurance Company, the United States Public Health Service, and the Milbank Memorial

Fund—did not use reliable state or national samples, or readily comparable methods, or control groups. Nevertheless, each of these studies reported an enormous and apparently increasing burden of sickness and disability resulting from chronic disease and injuries. Moreover, these studies described extensive disability among children and young adults.

The most important study of the "magnitude of the chronic disease problem in the United States" was the National Health Survey conducted by the Public Health Service in the winter of 1935–36. The survey was a "house-to-house canvass of some 800,000 families including 2,800,000 persons in 83 cities and 23 rural areas in 19 states." The response rate among families was 98 percent. The officials who designed the survey chose communities that were representative of national demography and selected participants at random. Wherever possible, the diagnoses reported by persons with disabilities or members of their families were checked with their personal physicians, 75 percent of whom responded to a questionnaire.[7]

The surveyors classified diseases as either acute or chronic. Acute conditions had "for the most part a fairly well defined onset and termination." Chronic diseases had "in general, a gradual, often imperceptible onset and sometimes periods of remission and recrudescence of symptoms."

Because of the difficulty of distinguishing between "normal health and the milder forms of ill-health," the officials who designed the survey used data about disability to create an operational definition of a "handicapping" condition. This was a "disabling illness which kept persons away from work, school or other usual pursuits for seven consecutive days or longer during the twelve months preceding the day of the canvass." The designers then expanded the definition to include "all confinement and hospital causes and deaths" and the traditional crippling disabilities of "orthopedic impairment, blindness and deafness."

The National Health Survey yielded four findings that had considerable significance for health policy for the rest of the twentieth century. The first finding was that more than one person in six in the United States had a disabling "chronic disease, orthopedic impairment or serious defect of hearing or vision."

The second conclusion was that each chronic disease had three potential levels of significance for individuals and for policy. The levels were prevalence, disability, and mortality. Rheumatism, for instance, was first in prevalence, second in disability, and only fourteenth as a cause of death. Tuberculosis had slipped to fifteenth in prevalence since the beginning of the century, but it remained of major significance as a cause of disability and death. In contrast, heart diseases and high blood pressure were "among the first five causes" in all three categories.

The third conclusion reinforced evidence from earlier morbidity surveys that "chronic disease is far from a problem of old age alone." Half of the persons for whom "chronic disease or impairments were reported were under 45 years of age, and over 70% of these persons were under 55 years."

Finally, the "frequency of chronic disabling illness and of the resulting problems of disability" was greatest among the lowest income groups. The average individual with a low income who had a disabling condition lost two to three times more days of work each year than a person with a comparable disability who had a higher income.

The Public Health Service officers who reported on the survey, led by George St. J. Perrott, emphasized its implications for policy. In an official publication, they said that the "total volume of chronic disease is growing. . . . [If] the greatest need for action in the field of public health is where the greatest saving of life and prevention of suffering can be made—then, without doubt, the chronic diseases deserve the attention they are getting." In a peer-reviewed journal, Perrott was more direct: the "inertia of the community" in most cities "in the face of this major health problem results from lack of awareness of its magnitude."[8]

Major chronic disease, Perrott and his colleagues insisted, could be prevented, postponed, or treated at early enough stages to enable people who had them, or early signs of them, to live longer and more productive lives. Their examples included cancer, diabetes, stroke, and heart disease.

The Priorities of Health Policy

The findings of the National Health Survey obviously did not transform health policy. This profound lack of influence is not surprising. It demonstrates yet again that data do not matter for policy unless people with compelling ideas and economic or professional stakes in those ideas act as effective interest groups. The survey used the best scientific methods of its time, was conducted at considerable public expense, had an enthusiastic response from interview subjects and their personal physicians, and had unambiguous results that were widely reported in public documents, professional journals, and the media. Moreover, subsequent surveys of disease and disability have generally confirmed and amplified the major conclusions of the National Health Survey.[9]

In the late 1930s, however, the only proponents of using the survey to change policy priorities were members of a loose coalition of clinical scientists, statisticians, physicians, and public health officials. The founders of that coalition, whom I describe in the next section of this chapter, were powerful and articulate individuals. But, as an interest group, they were no political match for other powerful people who had different priorities.

The bets on the future placed at the turn of the century by academic physicians and their allies in philanthropy and government paid off handsomely in the next few decades. Between the 1890s and the 1920s, these events, all of them familiar to readers of the history of medicine or social history, occurred throughout the United States:[10]

- The number and average size of hospitals increased, especially hospitals built and owned by charitable organizations, states, and cities.
- The equipment used in hospitals became increasingly sophisticated and expensive.
- The number of medical and surgical specialties and

subspecialties increased, and requirements for entering them became more rigorous.

- Reformers within medical education established more rigorous standards for admission and graduation and made achievement in laboratory research the major criterion for hiring, retaining, and promoting faculty.
- Teaching hospitals owned by or affiliated with the leading medical schools—and with formal and informal linkages to community hospitals, public and private clinics, and individual medical practitioners—became the dominant professional institutions providing medical care in their regions.
- Public health agencies in cities and states expanded in size and increased the scope of their authority for monitoring, preventing, and in many instances treating infectious diseases, especially among children.
- States, counties, and a few cities built and expanded facilities for treating mental illness and tuberculosis, while, in the largest cities, municipal hospitals became the major source of care for poor persons with chronic illness and injury.
- New state-mandated insurance programs of workmen's (now called workers') compensation provided income, treatment, and rehabilitative services for injuries in the workplace and acute sickness caused by environmental toxins.

These events exemplified the priorities of American health policy: increasing the supply of facilities and professionals providing acute care, expanding community-based public health services to control infectious disease, and ameliorating the financial consequences of injury in the workplace and of acute occupational illness. The events also reinforced those priorities by greatly increasing the number of people whose livelihoods depended on existing health policy and by creating a vast amount of what economists call sunk capital.

The most prestigious institutions of the health sector were teaching hospitals, medical schools, and research laboratories. Teaching hospitals allocated most of their resources to treating acute episodes of illness among inpatients. Medical schools educated practitioners to value most highly and to be most adept at intervention in acute conditions. Research laboratories, with a few notable exceptions, continued until the 1940s to emphasize the investigation of infectious diseases, in part because of scientific fashion, but also because of the presumed intellectual difficulty of research on chronic disease.

Most policy makers regarded the management of chronic illness and disability as mainly a problem for people with the lowest incomes. The needs of the chronically sick or injured poor would be met by state mental hospitals, by the sanatoria and general hospitals run by city and county government, and by workmen's compensation.

When public health officials and most physicians in private practice considered the problem of preventing chronic disease at all, they usually dismissed it. Preventing most chronic disease was a private, not a public, responsibility; people should not have advice about private matters pressed on them. The great exception was, of course, chronic infectious disease, notably tuberculosis and syphilis, though voluntary associations also issued public information about the danger signs for cancer and mental illness. These afflictions seemed to be preventable, or at least they could be defended against by methods derived from the study of infection in laboratories and teaching hospitals. Affluent people should receive preventive advice from their personal physicians. Prevention was more difficult for people in the poorer social classes, who, public health officials assumed, were more resistant to sound advice than people who had more money. Poorer people required special, segregated preventive campaigns, sponsored by public or philanthropic agencies.

The advocates of reform in health care finance shared most of the priorities of their antagonists. They simply wanted to improve access to hospital and medical services for people with acute conditions in the working and lower-middle classes. The most doctrinaire reformers proposed that insurance funds for acute care be created, that everyone be required to purchase coverage from them in order to create large pools, and that they should be managed by public agencies. Beginning in the late 1920s, they also endorsed the reorganization of medical practice into groups of generalists and specialists. They were vilified and consistently defeated in their efforts to make national and state policy, mainly by coalitions of organized medicine and the business community.[11] But they agreed with their adversaries about the need for more and better facilities, better-trained specialists, and additional funding for research.

Beginning in the early 1930s, an intensely pragmatic group of advocates for health care finance reform came up with a plan that they hoped would be satisfactory to leaders of business and medicine and at the same time would allay working people's anxiety about paying for expensive hospital stays for acute conditions. The vehicles for this accommodation of interests were voluntary, nonprofit, prepaid hospital plans, soon called Blue Cross. During and after World War II, these Blue Cross plans, now joined by commercial health insurance companies, proliferated as benefits were tied to employment. They did so because federal policy excluded their cost from the taxable earnings of individuals and corporations. For the first time, the risks of a significant number of Americans were being pooled in order to avoid the catastrophic costs of illness.

Like most specialized physicians and hospital managers, most of the health finance reformers, whether doctrinaire or pragmatic, regarded the management of chronic illness as a distraction from their priorities. Advocates of state or national health insurance wanted everyone to be required by law to be covered for acute services. These reformers were most eager to ensure that working people would have access to private physicians, who could admit patients to private and nonprofit hospitals. The reformers associated chronic disabling illness with the charity care offered by public hospitals and their clinics or with the indignities and irritations of workers' compensation. Similarly, the organizers of the first Blue Cross plans gave priority to setting affordable subscription fees (the nonprofit phrase for premiums) that would cover the devastating cost of acute illness. An early advertising slogan of the new plan in New York City was "three cents a day."

This appealingly low fee for subscribers nearly caused the plan to declare bankruptcy. In 1939, to avoid bankruptcy, the plan was forced to drop enrollees who were not employed and to reduce coverage for normal pregnancies.

A series of political events in 1938 exemplify these generalizations about the priorities of health policy reformers. In 1937, President Franklin D. Roosevelt appointed a federal interagency committee—chaired by George Perrott, who had recently directed the National Health Survey—to prepare a National Health Program. The program had four parts: federal subsidies for hospital construction; grants to the states to help them pay for services to low-income pregnant mothers and young children; direct federal payments to support blind persons, crippled children, and persons with temporary disabilities; and financial support for states that wanted to organize programs of compulsory health insurance. The American Medical Association declared that it would support the first three parts of the program, but only if the Roosevelt administration abandoned its tentative support for state compulsory insurance plans. Reformers within and outside government believed, however, that they had sufficient political support to persuade Congress to pass the entire program. During a national radio broadcast on the Columbia network, for instance, Surgeon General Thomas Parran called the program, and the National Health Conference convened to launch it, the "greatest event in medical science which has happened in our time."[12]

Two intertwined interest groups—the American Hospital Association and its affiliate, the new association of Blue Cross plans—proposed a compromise on health insurance to the federal interagency committee. The spokesman for the hospitals and prepaid plans, C. Rufus Rorem, understood the problems created for health policy by chronic illness. Six years earlier, Rorem had explained that these prepaid plans (soon to be called Blue Cross plans) would limit reimbursement for hospital care for each episode of illness, so that the plans and the hospitals would be protected "against large expense for chronic or incurable disease." Because most voluntary prepaid groups were too small to cover chronic disease, the "proportion of individuals" in any insured group "suffering from these problems" would not be uniform. Therefore, Rorem reasoned, payment for treatment of chronic disease "should be made the responsibility of the entire community," the largest possible pool over which to spread risks, and should be subsidized with public funds.[13]

In 1938, Rorem combined the principle of community-wide risk pooling with a new method of paying for hospital and medical services for people with low incomes. Moreover, his proposal was acceptable to the AMA. The federal government would encourage cities to establish prepayment plans for hospital service that would be offered in the open wards of public and voluntary hospitals. These plans would also cover physicians' fees. People receiving care in the wards would now be treated by private physicians as well as by interns and residents. The working poor would, in exchange for regular payments, no longer be means-tested for hospitalization at public expense. Cities and states, perhaps with some federal participation, "might subsidize a portion of a plan for those who are unable to pay." In sum, poor people with chronic disabling conditions and private physicians would gain. City governments would save money or break even.

In a closed session of the committee, the civil servant representing the federal Social Security Board, Isadore S. Falk, attacked Rorem's proposal as inferior to comprehensive compulsory health insurance based on state or national risk pools and subsidized with federal and state funds. Falk was convinced that enrollment in the Blue Cross group hospital plans had peaked and might even decline in the near future. He did not address the problem of chronic illness. Neither did Perrott, who apparently kept his two official roles in separate compartments.

The committee recommended against accepting the compromises offered by any of the interest groups. In the absence of consensus among the groups, and wary of the hostility of the AMA, President Roosevelt merely transmitted the recommendations of the interagency committee to Congress, where, lacking his endorsement, they expired. In the politics of the time, it was more important to uphold principles sacred to both the advocates of compulsory insurance and the leaders of dominant provider interest groups than to solve the problems of access to health care for low-income people. The growing burden of chronic illness was simply an incidental issue.

Mobilizing a Constituency for Chronic Disabling Disease

For some prominent people in health affairs in the 1920s and 1930s, however, the burden of chronic illness was the major unresolved issue of health policy. The advocates of higher priority for chronic illness in health policy were employees of prestigious institutions. Their advocacy was politely phrased and encountered noncomprehension more often than principled resistance. Unlike the clashes between organized medicine and advocates of national health insurance, this story received no attention in the mass media and has been ignored by most historians of health and social policy.

Six men organized a coalition to advocate higher priority for chronic illness in health policy. These men were Alfred E. Cohn, George Bigelow, Ernst Boas, Louis Dublin, Alan Gregg, and Sigmund S. Goldwater. They worked separately and together, conducting research, writing in professional journals, teaching, and serving on committees and boards. Two of them, Bigelow and Goldwater, both physicians, held prominent public positions. Bigelow served as commissioner of health for the Commonwealth of Massachusetts. Goldwater was superintendent of Mount Sinai Hospital and commissioner of health and, later, commissioner of hospitals for New York City. In the last years of his life, he became the chief executive of the largest Blue Cross plan in the country. Cohn was a clinical scientist at the Rockefeller Institute for medical research. Boas was chief physician at the Montefiore Hospital and held an academic position at the College of Physicians and Surgeons of Columbia University. Dublin, trained in biology, was chief statistician for the Metropolitan Life Insurance Company. Gregg, a physician educated at Harvard, was a senior official of the Rockefeller Foundation.[14]

From the 1920s to the 1940s, Cohn was the leading advocate of higher priority for research on chronic disease. He recalled in 1953 that he first became aware of the importance of chronic disease in 1922, when Royal S. Copeland, then New York City commissioner of health and soon to be a United States senator, published newspaper articles claiming that death rates from infectious diseases of childhood had been falling for many years. By 1926, Cohn was ready to challenge the priorities of medical research, most of which was funded by foundations, principally the various Rockefeller philanthropies. Using published statistics, he demonstrated that organic heart disease had two underlying causes—not one, as most physicians and scientists believed. Rheumatic fever, an infection, accounted for most heart disease among people under the age of forty. For older people, the principal cause was arteriosclerosis, a chronic degenerative condition; because of this condition, the "rate of so-called heart disease is high and is constantly mounting."

By the early 1930s, Cohn was exerting some influence on the priorities of medical science. A 1933 survey conducted under Boas's auspices for a consortium of New York foundations and service organizations reported that about half the diseases under study at the Rockefeller Institute's research hospital were chronic conditions. Two years later, Simon Flexner, who had helped shape the policy priorities of the turn of the century, retired as founding director of the institute. His successor, Herbert Gasser, shared Cohen's priorities. Announcing Gasser's appointment to the press, John D. Rockefeller, Jr., said that the "time has now come" to study chronic disease by more intensive "investigation of fundamental life processes at the level of the cell and its constituents."

Cohn's influence extended beyond the Rockefeller Institute. In publications and correspondence, he insisted that each chronic disease is the result of a biological process that should be studied in detail from onset to death. In 1935—speaking to fellow board members of a new foundation that sponsored research on aging— he said that "new armies of destruction . . . the heart diseases, cancer, diseases of the kidney" for instance, required changes in the concept of the hospital. These changes would include extending the "arm of the outpatient department . . . to the home or the patient's place of occupation." In the emerging world of research and medical practice, moreover, there was no "sharp or clear distinction . . . between normal and pathological."[15] The same year, Cohn collaborated with Goldwater, Gregg, and Dublin to establish the first clinical research center anywhere to give priority to the study of chronic disease. The center was part of a new municipal hospital that treated patients with chronic disease on Welfare (now Roosevelt) Island in New York's East River.

Boas was a more visible public figure than Cohn, because he addressed medical and general audiences about the broad implications of chronic illness for medical practice and social policy. His base, Montefiore Hospital, was one of very few voluntary institutions established to care for persons with chronic diseases. Boas challenged two principles of the contemporary health policy consensus. The first was that hospitals should be arrayed in hierarchies, at the top of which were teaching institutions providing acute medical and surgical care. He insisted that persons with chronic disease should be treated, often for long periods of time, either in dedicated units in general hospitals or in separate hospitals. Hospitals that specialized in treating patients with chronic illness should, moreover, be affiliated with medical schools. Second, Boas challenged the principle that health policy should be separated from other social policies, especially for the elderly. For example, he described the most important priorities for health policy as old-age pensions, sickness insurance, and replacement of the remaining almshouses with state hospitals for chronic disease. Boas, like his colleagues in the new network advocating higher priority for chronic illness, repeatedly insisted that these afflictions were neither incurable nor results of the "natural decrepitude of old age."

In 1941, in what seems to have been the first textbook on treating a variety of chronic diseases, Boas linked his principles to general medical practice. He told his readers that because their "young patients are far healthier than they were in former generations . . . many more of them grow to middle age and become afflicted in their mature years with circulatory disorders, diabetes, chronic 'rheumatism,' cancer or some of the other so-called degenerative chronic diseases." These diseases are "insidious in their onset, chronic in their course, and lead to irreversible changes in the human organism." Treatment for these conditions is "much more complex than [for] the acute infectious diseases." Moreover, the "practicing physician will become the chief agent of preventive medicine in the field of chronic diseases."[16]

Louis Dublin, chief statistician of the nation's largest life insurance company, sorrowfully concluded in the mid-1920s that the growing burden of chronic illness contradicted the fundamental assumption of health policy since the 1890s: the assumption that medical progress against disease would be continuous. In 1929, for example, he worried in a private memorandum that mortality after age forty-five "apparently has gotten worse" in the past decade. Contemporary conditions "are apparently wiping out the gains from fewer cases of infection." In 1931, Dublin decided that the incidence of cancer had reached epidemic proportions.

Dublin was frustrated by the consensus on the priorities of health policy. In 1934, when he worked with Goldwater to design the first benefits contract for the Associated Hospital Service, the organization that would become New York's Blue Cross, he tried but failed to get agreement to include coverage for venereal disease. He reluctantly yielded to Goldwater's reasoning that chronic disease had to be excluded from coverage because the cost would be excessive if it was spread only over a risk pool made up of volunteers in one city. But even this compromise held too many business risks for his superiors at Metropolitan Life. Wary of any involvement with insurance for illness, they did not permit him to serve on the board of the Associated Hospital Service.

Most public health officers in the 1920s and 1930s regarded chronic disease as a private matter, just as Boas had said. George Bigelow of Massachusetts was almost the sole exception to the prevailing opinion that chronic disease lay outside the authority of government agencies. When he sent a questionnaire about policy for chronic disease to other state and provincial health officers in the United States and Canada, all but three of them replied that "they were doing nothing about adult hygiene or chronic disease. . . . Many hoped they never would."

Bigelow himself had until recently been ambivalent about the place of chronic disease in public health policy. In 1925, he disagreed with a resolution adopted by the American Public Health Association, at the insistence of academics rather than public officials. The resolution asserted that chronic disease was a legitimate area of public health practice. In Bigelow's view, chronic diseases were a "purely personal matter," not a responsibility of the community. By 1929, he had changed his mind. When a charitable organization invited Dublin to Boston to speak about communicable diseases, Bigelow persuaded him to talk instead about "chronic disease . . . the most important medical social problem facing us." After Dublin's speech, he and Bigelow lobbied a prominent member of the audience, Ray Lyman Wilbur, the former dean of medicine and president of Stanford University, who was serving as President Hoover's secretary of the interior (the Public Health Service was then assigned to the Interior Department). Wilbur had recently been selected to chair a Committee on the Costs of Medical Care financed by major national foundations, including Rockefeller, Rosenwald, and Milbank. But Bigelow and Dublin failed to persuade Wilbur of the overwhelming importance of chronic disease for policy.

Bigelow soon organized the first comprehensive public program to diagnose, treat, and conduct epidemiological research on cancer. His ambivalence about the appropriateness of public health intervention to detect and treat chronic disease was an unexpectedly effective political tactic. The Massachusetts Health Department appeared to be dragged into its cancer program by the legislature, with the cautious support of most leaders of the medical profession and enthusiastic advocacy by a few prominent medical researchers at teaching hospitals affiliated with Harvard.

In 1933, Bigelow and Herbert L. Lombard published an account of the Massachusetts cancer program that became a handbook for subsequent chronic disease surveys and control programs. Abandoning his remaining ambivalence about the importance of chronic disease in public health practice, Bigelow insisted that the "outstanding sickness and health problem of the present day is the control of chronic diseases of the middle-aged."

Alan Gregg, director of the Division of Medical Sciences of the Rockefeller Foundation, was another prominent member of the coalition advocating greater priority for chronic illness. In 1935, he persuaded the foundation's trustees to establish a new program of research in the sciences underlying psychiatry. Unlike infectious disease, he wrote, chronic diseases, including mental illness, were "disorders of the organism as a whole." Understanding the causes of these diseases required fundamental knowledge that went beyond the study of "bodily disorders caused by parasites and bacteria, viruses, poisons, inadequate nutrition and hereditary defect." Three years later, Gregg recommended that the board give a research grant to the new clinical research center for chronic disease on Welfare Island. That was the first of almost a decade of research grants to the center.

Sigmund S. Goldwater was a reluctant innovator in policy for chronic disease. As the most prominent hospital administrator of his generation, he had defended the prevailing assumption among his peers that care for chronically ill patients was the "function of public hospitals." In the mid-1930s, however, when he served Mayor Fiorello La Guardia as commissioner of hospitals and chaired the committee established by the United Hospital Fund to organize New York's first voluntary health insurance program, Goldwater began to change his opinion. Voluntary hospitals were admitting vast numbers of persons with chronic illness and seeing even more of them in their outpatient clinics. Public hospitals were increasingly being staffed and equipped to treat acutely ill patients. As commissioner of hospitals, and then from 1939 to 1942 as chief executive of Blue Cross, Goldwater spent the last years of his life stimulating partnerships between public and voluntary institutions to address chronic disease.

The Politics of Incremental Accommodation

In the early 1940s, none of the six leading advocates on behalf of policy for chronic illness would have claimed more than modest influence on the consensus about the priorities of health policy.

Although they had participated in exemplary projects or major shifts in priority in particular institutions, they knew very well that much more needed to be done.

The process by which health policy in the United States would accommodate chronic illness during the remainder of the century had, however, been established. Instead of sudden or even gradual reform, any changes that took place would be incremental and often unacknowledged. Leaders of public and private organizations and representatives of powerful interest groups in health care quietly helped to accommodate particular policies to the epidemiological situation, simultaneously insisting that the overall priorities of health policy were absolutely correct.

The behavior of physicians and hospital managers exemplified the politics of incremental accommodation. Growing numbers of patients with chronic illness populated the practices of physicians and used an increasing proportion of available hospital beds. The disabling conditions these patients presented required management over the long course, as described by Alfred Cohen and the investigators he influenced; the clinical methods urged by Ernst Boas and his disciples were used to treat these patients. But the prestige of particular medical specialists and hospitals would for the next half century be determined by their prowess in addressing acute episodes of illness.

The accommodation of policy to chronic illness was gradual and fragmented. Only in retrospect does it seem to have been inexorable. A history of accommodation could be written about every area of health policy: research, patient care, education, and financing. In the late 1930s, Alfred Cohn noted that his colleagues in research were "struggling to discover if the strain of caring for chronic disease can be relieved," though they were not yet doing so "very consciously." Blue Cross did not explicitly cover treatment for chronic disease during Goldwater's presidency. But corporate policy began to change shortly after his death when surgery for pulmonary tuberculosis and treatment for congenital anomalies and venereal diseases were included as standard benefits for the first time.

Commercial health insurance also accommodated chronic illness, but more slowly and sometimes with strange logic. Dublin, for instance, representing Metropolitan Life's official opinion rather than his own, said in 1942 that chronic diseases "affect only a small portion of our policyholders," when he explained the company's withdrawal from the consortium funding the research center established by Goldwater on Welfare Island.

Accommodation was also evident in federal health policy. Until 1933, the program providing medical assistance to veterans of World War I for illnesses unconnected to their service was the only federal program of direct payment that included chronic illness. Beginning that year, however, federal funds for economic relief programs were used to pay physicians to treat persons with chronic conditions. In 1935, the Social Security Act authorized federal grants to the states for assistance to crippled children and, more important, stimulated the establishment of nonprofit and proprietary nursing homes by stipulating that federal aid to the blind and the needy would be given only when they lived in their own homes or in private institutions.

Federal research policy also began to accord higher priority to the study of chronic disease. In 1932, preparing testimony to the House Committee on Appropriations, Surgeon General Parran decided that "we ought to begin our study of the degenerative diseases of adult life and take up first the cause of deaths from heart disease." By 1935, chronic disease was high on an internal PHS priority list for spending the research funds appropriated in the Social Security Act of 1935.

But accommodation also had limits within the federal government. A 1936 report on research in progress at the National Institutes of Health contained four pages of studies on infectious disease but only three lines on chronic disease. Similarly, in 1937, the surgeon general was less enthusiastic than members of Congress and editors of leading newspapers about the bill passed that year to create a new National Cancer Institute.

Accommodation to the pressures of chronic illness accelerated during World War II, especially in hospital and research policy, areas in which there was bipartisan political agreement on the need for additional federal subsidy. During the negotiations that

resulted in subsidies for hospital construction under the Hill-
Burton Act of 1946, a coalition of hospital leaders, supported by
officials of foundations and federal agencies, revised the consensus about the role of voluntary hospitals. The new consensus on
hospital services accommodated the older theory of hospital planning to the growing burden of chronic illness. According to the
theory of hierarchical regionalism promulgated in the first thirty
years of the century, physicians should refer patients from less to
more sophisticated settings for treatment of acute conditions that
threatened their health and lives. In the revised planning theory of
the 1940s, each level of a regional hierarchy should now include
facilities to treat persons with chronic disease, in general as well
as special hospitals. These revisions were proposed by the American Hospital Association, the Public Health Service, and various
state planning commissions.

Wartime priorities temporarily interrupted the redirection of
medical research to give higher priority to the study of chronic
illness. During the war, research on illness and injury was
managed by a federal Office of Scientific Research and Develop-
ment (OSRD) through its Committee on Medical Research. The
committee awarded several thousand contracts to investigate war-
related problems, mainly studies of prevention and treatment for
infection and response to traumatic injuries.

These contracts were the basis for what became the extramural
grants program of the National Institutes of Health. First, in what
appeared to be a technical amendment to the statute reauthoriz-
ing the Public Health Service in 1943, Congress permitted grants
to be made for research on other diseases than cancer. But officials of the Bureau of the Budget were reluctant to ask Congress
to fund the new grant program. In 1945, the leaders of the National Institutes of Health bypassed the bureau and awarded
grants to selected wartime contractors, using surplus OSRD funds
to make the initial awards.[17] Projects begun as wartime procure-
ment of practical work on infection and trauma thus became the
basis of a postwar research program of investigator-initiated
grants focused on the biology of chronic disease. At the research
center founded by Goldwater, Gregg, Cohn, and Dublin on Wel-

fare Island in New York, for example, a group led by James Shannon resumed its work in renal physiology, having abandoned it to study malaria during the war. Shannon and others in his group, notably Julius Axelrod, Robert Berliner, and Thomas Kennedy, soon moved to NIH, where they would for a generation be prominent leaders.[18]

New strategies to promote research on chronic disease emerged during and immediately after the war. Albert Lasker, who had sought advice from Alfred Cohn since the 1920s, made a grant to the American Cancer Society to raise the priority it accorded to research. His wife, Mary (guided by Mary Switzer, a close friend who served in the senior management first of the Public Health Service and then of its parent agency), lobbied to create new national institutes for mental health and heart disease and to expand the overall research budget.[19]

By the late 1940s, a bipartisan coalition in Congress and among interest groups was successfully promoting research on chronic disease. In the absence of a politically effective coalition for reform in financing health services, national chronic disease policy became primarily research policy. During and immediately after the war, however, pressure increased on voluntary insurance plans to expand coverage for chronic illness. The number of subscribers to both Blue Cross/Blue Shield and commercial insurance plans had grown. Many of these new subscribers, and the unions representing them, wanted more comprehensive coverage. But broader coverage would make insurance more expensive unless the costs of treatment for illness could be spread over much larger risk pools than the average employer group or the members of a community who volunteered to be covered.

In the absence of larger risk pools similar to those used in most of Western Europe, broader coverage by voluntary insurance would cause premiums to rise. Higher premiums created three problems for the insurance industry. They would drive away the healthiest subscribers, thus causing more upward pressure on premiums. They would make the more comprehensive plans the most expensive, thus causing employee groups with the healthiest members to purchase insurance from competitors with lower prices. Finally, and most important from the point of view of both Blue Cross and commercial insurers, higher premiums for more comprehensive policies could make compulsory insurance, with large risk pools organized or regulated by government, more attractive to voters and hence, through pressure from unions and consumer interest groups, to state legislators and members of Congress.

A few leaders of Blue Cross wanted to make coverage both more extensive and more comprehensive by combining public and private insurance. Rufus Rorem, for example, updated his 1938 scheme for prepaid care in the wards of public and large voluntary hospitals. In New York, Goldwater's successor as chief executive of Blue Cross recommended that state government pay the cost of voluntary insurance for the poor and that the state and employers share the costs of insurance for workers with low wages. His proposal died, even though it was endorsed by the Medical Society of the County of New York and the science editor of the *New York Times*.[20]

Such schemes had few supporters in postwar politics. Business leaders and their trade associations identified the "voluntary way" with the "American way." Organized medicine moved further to the political right, tolerating only the expansion of the National Institutes of Health, the passage and funding of the Hill-Burton Act for constructing acute general hospitals, and health care for veterans as acceptable federal actions in civilian health policy.

Limits of Accommodation:
The Cortisone Story

Americans by 1950 had the best-funded research on chronic disease; the most extensive program to construct general hospitals, long-term care facilities, and medical schools; and the least comprehensive health insurance of any industrial country. At the same time, they had enormous optimism about their future health, even as the burden of chronic disabling illness increased. For many of these people, the health policy priorities of the turn of the century were still valid. Americans who continued to endorse these priorities included many health professionals, journalists, and, according to public opinion polls, ordinary citizens. New cures and techniques for diagnosis emerged from laboratories, to be tested in teaching hospitals and then disseminated to practicing physicians. The new and enlarged hospitals being built in every community were sources of great civic pride. As a result of prosperity and the spread of voluntary insurance, semiprivate rooms were quickly replacing the crowded, smelly, and noisy open hospital wards. The country seemed to need many more physicians, and by the late 1940s states were appropriating large sums to expand and create medical schools to produce them.[21]

Many people talked about chronic illness. Surgeon General Leonard Scheele, who succeeded Parran in 1948, was a specialist in research on cancer; he made chronic illness the highest priority of the Public Health Service. But few people in medicine, philanthropy, or government agreed with Alfred Cohn that research agencies should give more emphasis to investigating the etiology or the natural history and epidemiology of chronic disease. Even fewer agreed with Boas that both the treatment of patients with chronic disease and social policies were the results of misguided priorities.

The prevailing optimism, despite the increasing incidence and prevalence of chronic disease, was expressed at a 1951 conference sponsored by every major national medical, public health, and public welfare organization, as well as the Public Health Service. Self-congratulation was in order about preventing chronic disease, the subject of the conference. David Seegal, the current research director of the pioneer clinical research center established by Goldwater and his colleagues in the 1930s, took for granted "our mastery over the acute infectious diseases, except those of small viral origin." We are, he predicted, "on the threshold of the Golden Age of achievement" in the prevention of chronic disease.[22]

The Nobel Prize jury in Stockholm had agreed with him just six months earlier, when it awarded the prize in medicine or physiol-

ogy to two Americans and a Swiss for research on the cortical
steroid that seemed to cause remission of the symptoms of rheumatoid arthritis. The new substance, called Cortisone by its pro-
prietor, the Merck Company, had been revealed to the public at
a special meeting for scientists and the press at the Mayo Clinic in
April 1949.[23]

Cortisone seemed to prove the correctness of the priorities of
twentieth-century health policy. The potency of the substance had
been discovered in the laboratory by biochemist Edward Kendall.
Philip Hench, the principal investigator, had tested its clinical
potential on patients at the world-famous Mayo Clinic. At the
press briefing, Hench showed a film of patients before and after
treatment. The "miracle of Cortisone" was displayed first in *Life*
magazine and then in the nation's newspapers. Surgeon General
Scheele, with Hench beside him, described the miracle and
showed the film to a committee of Congress. Even President Truman became involved in the search for ways to find a botanical
source of Cortisone or to produce more of it from animals. The
press and many medical scientists declared that the miracle of
Cortisone was proof that the methods used to triumph over infections could be transferred to the problem of chronic disease. Cortisone was but the most recent in a short but promising list of new
therapies that began with the sulfa drugs and now included peni-
cillin and streptomycin. The Public Health Service immediately
asked Congress to create a National Institute of Arthritis.

The vexing problem of access to Cortisone was its supply, not
its price. Many people assumed that supply, not demand, would
be the major problem of policy for access to care for other chronic
diseases in the future.

The next stage in the history of Cortisone as a remedy for
rheumatoid arthritis did not have the same political effects. In
1951, extensive randomized clinical trials of Cortisone began in
the United Kingdom. Even before the trials started, a few medical
scientists in the United States had questioned Hench's methodol-
ogy and noted that Cortisone had painful side effects in some
patients and did not cause remission of symptoms in others. In
1954, the results of the trials revealed that Cortisone was about as

effective as aspirin in treating patients with rheumatoid arthritis. Nevertheless, Cortisone continued for years to be cited as proof that the policies aimed at curing infection were appropriate for treating chronic disease.

Cortisone, in sum, is a metaphor for health policy that looked to the past for its priorities while the people who made it and those who gained the most personal income and prestige from it believed that they were using the best new science to create better health in the future. Cortisone also exemplifies the linkage of power and illness. Government appropriations and the insurance premiums paid by employers and employees supported the grandest ambitions of medical scientists, specialist physicians, hospital managers, and manufacturers of pharmaceutical drugs. Almost all of these powerful people also chose to give priority to the acute phases of the chronic diseases that afflicted the people. The paradox of health policy rested on the disjunction between belief and information.

The Cortisone story reveals the limits of the accommodation of health policy to chronic illness. Cortisone made many people, within and outside health affairs, optimistic about the future. It provided them, they believed, with a model for future policy. At the same time, the partial accommodation to chronic disease in the organization and financing of health services meant that the burden of cost and insecurity for individual Americans would unavoidably increase in the future. Cortisone symbolized health policies that could solve the problems of supplying research, manpower, facilities, and pharmaceuticals but that could address demand for health care only by driving costs ever higher.

3

The Health Policy
Compromise, 1950-1975

By 1950, the most influential people in American health affairs had rationalized to their own satisfaction the paradox of health policy—that is, the mismatch between the allocation of resources and human need. Facing only the facts and interest groups they found compelling, leaders of public agencies and private institutions accommodated chronic illness and its consequent disability within policy that had been intended to address acute episodes of illness. For the next quarter century, these decision makers and their successors continued the pattern of policy making that had proved successful in attracting resources to the health sector and enhancing the prestige of its leaders. I call the history of these events the "health policy compromise." It is the story of a negotiated balance of competing interests that persisted for many years.

In the third quarter of the century, most of the people who made health policy or sought to influence it still insisted that the health status of Americans would improve mainly as a result of scientific and economic progress. There was a strong consensus on the need to subsidize medical research and increase investment in facilities and personnel. The most intense disagreements were about how to organize services and provide insurance coverage for people with acute diseases. As in the previous quarter century, however, policy makers accommodated incrementally to the problems of caring for people with chronic disabling illness.

As the amount of money in the health sector increased, so did conflict among groups representing the interests of payers, consumers, and service providers. People with stakes in health politics included legislators and executives in federal, state, and local government; officials of trade associations and labor unions; advocates for children, the elderly, and persons with particular diseases and disabilities; and leaders of organizations of practicing physicians, medical scientists, and managers of hospitals and other facilities. Representatives of these groups negotiated what was, in effect, a compromise on the priorities of spending for health care. They described the compromise in an array of laws, regulations, and agreements between business and labor about wages and benefits. Health care was to be financed by direct public subsidy; tax expenditures (that is, government revenue forgone as a result of exclusions, deductions, and exemptions from income tax); employers, employees, retirees, and their families; and private investment. The areas of policy that were part of the compromise included research, investment in manpower and facilities, responsibility for prevention and public health, and the organizing and financing of personal health services.

It was a compromise by default. To most contemporaries who participated in or paid close attention to the struggles among interest groups, each agreement about policy was not a component of a stable compromise but was, instead, a victory or defeat in an ongoing struggle. The most self-aware of the compromisers were public officials and executives of Blue Cross and Blue Shield plans, who worked to create a mix of social and market-driven insurance for health services.

The terms of what turned out to be a persisting compromise were as follows. The federal government subsidized most medical research. Foundations and charities dedicated to particular diseases made smaller contributions to research. The states, the federal government, and private investors provided capital for building and renovating hospitals and research laboratories. The states took major responsibility for financing the facilities and faculty to educate physicians and other professionals. The states also were primarily responsible for financing care for persons with mental illness and mental retardation and for the surveillance, preventive, and regulatory activities of public health agencies. Most people were insured for hospital and some physician care through their employment. Health insurance for the elderly was organized under Social Security as a combination of social insurance, paid by all taxpayers, and voluntary supplemental coverage. The poor and the uninsured received care through federal and state programs, mainly in hospitals and clinics subsidized by state and local taxes.

Two powerful and antagonistic groups, New Deal liberals (proponents of an expanded welfare state) and market-oriented conservatives (proponents of freer markets in capital, labor, and goods), were most troubled by this compromise. The New Deal liberals, many of whom were associated with large industrial unions, complained that the compromise poorly served most persons with low incomes. They advocated national health insurance with a single governmental payer. The conservatives, many of whom acted through associations of manufacturing and business executives, complained that the federal government and many of the states were overregulating health care providers and taxing individuals and corporations too heavily in order to provide services for the poor. They advocated greater reliance on economic competition to provide health services to individuals and families.

Both the New Deal liberals and the conservatives (many of whom preferred to be called classical liberals) assumed that much of the health policy made in the quarter century after 1950 was temporary. Most of the New Dealers and their political heirs assumed that national health insurance was imminent, especially during the decade after 1965. Many conservatives predicted that Americans' deep-seated distrust of intrusive central government would soon lead to policies that were responsive to a new coalition of voters, who preferred private sector to welfare state solutions. Advocates of each competing ideology also assumed for many years that prosperity would help their cause. In the 1950s and

1960s, liberals claimed that a compassionate, increasingly centralized state could distribute the surplus created by American abundance wisely and to the satisfaction of most of the public. Conservatives, in contrast, believed during these years that the wealth created by the economic growth that accompanied freer markets would benefit members of every social class.

Despite these ideological differences and the irritation that leaders of the interest groups expressed routinely about each other, most Americans—or at least most political leaders, business executives, and union officials—accepted the health policy compromise. One source of satisfaction was that the compromise achieved widespread security against the costs of most hospital stays. By the 1950s, almost all working people, and members of their immediate families, had insurance that paid most of the cost of hospitalization. A decade later, federal legislation extended this security to the elderly and to most of the poor.

Throughout the century, most people feared the costs of hospitalization for acute conditions more than they did the costs of care for chronic illness and disability. The phrase *catastrophic illness* has had a double meaning for a long time. Most Americans paid the costs of managing their own and their dependents' chronic illnesses out of current income or from savings and from the uncompensated work of wives, mothers, and sisters. Long-established public programs paid many of the costs of care for the poor who suffered chronic physical or mental illness. Moreover, most people—whether their politics were liberal, centrist, or conservative—agreed about the importance of conducting more biomedical research and increasing the supply of health professionals and facilities for treatment and care. People disagreed not about the desirability of these activities but instead about appropriate levels of federal, state, and private sector spending and influence.

The health policy compromise of the third quarter of the century became more expensive and, as a result, increasingly disappointing to almost everyone who consumed, provided, paid for, or regulated care. Demand for health services increased, mainly because of expectations created by new medical technology and because of an increasing number of elderly people in the population. But demand also grew because of the increasing supply of physicians and other professionals who were eager to meet it and were handsomely reimbursed by private insurance, Medicare, and Medicaid.

The cost of managing chronic illness became a more important concern for public policy in the 1970s than it had been in the 1950s and the 1960s. Most of these costs continued to be paid by individuals, families, and, as a last resort, state and local government. But the cost of chronic care was increasing as a result of advancing medical technology and demographic changes that made it necessary for individuals to pay strangers for work previously contributed by relatives and neighbors.

The Supply of Services for Chronic Disabling Illness

A great deal more was said than done about chronic disabling illness in the third quarter of the century. National commissions appointed by government agencies, foundations, and interest groups repeatedly documented the scope of the problem and held conferences to recommend policy. Agencies of state and local government spent more time and money regulating and subsidizing nursing homes and home health care agencies; preventing cancer, hypertension, and other chronic conditions; and caring for persons who were mentally ill and developmentally disabled. During the 1950s, coalitions of physicians, business and union leaders, and university officials, in their efforts to persuade state officials to establish new medical schools, routinely pointed to the increasing prevalence of chronic disease among the elderly.[1] This apparent concern for chronic disease was, however, tactical, a means to other ends. Interest groups eager to maintain the priority accorded to acute care in health services used the burden of chronic illness to achieve their goals. Nowhere was this tactic more evident than in medical and hospital practice and in the behavior of medical educators.

An unexpected result of World War II was that an increasing

number of physicians now specialized in the care of patients with particular chronic diseases. Between the world wars, as Kenneth Ludmerer writes, the "great triumph of graduate medical education . . . was that almost all trainees entered general practice."[2] By the mid-1950s, however, specialists outnumbered generalists, and the ratio continued to increase. The higher rank and safer duty accorded certified specialists in the military during the war helped to stimulate this reversal of priority between generalists and specialists. The reversal was accelerated by payments under the G.I. Bill to physicians who entered specialty training after their military service.

In the late 1940s and early 1950s, thousands of former general physicians emerged from residencies and fellowships in teaching hospitals as specialists in treating the acute consequences of chronic diseases. Most of them received fees from patients or their insurers for each service they provided; and they were paid more for performing procedures, both diagnostic and therapeutic, than for assessing information and advising their patients. The payment system thus reinforced the clinical priorities of hospital-based residency training. Higher payments had historically been made to physicians who performed time-consuming procedures that invaded the human body because these individuals required special training and could see fewer patients than could their colleagues.

Hospitals also gave priority to intervention, even though their administrators assured state planning officials that they were increasingly attentive to patients with chronic illness. From the 1950s on, hospital managers became preoccupied with acquiring new equipment for intensive care and surgery. They hoped that this new equipment would enable them to attract physicians, and thus the physicians' patients, to their medical staffs. Blue Cross plans subsidized this competition among hospitals by amortizing the cost of new equipment in the audited payments they made to hospitals for each patient day. In their billings to commercial insurers, hospitals included as many of the costs of technology as they could get away with. The Blues and the insurance companies passed these subsidies on to employers and employees in premiums. Although the Hill-Burton Act was amended in 1954 to permit hospitals to build outpatient departments, nursing homes, and rehabilitation facilities, the new federal subsidies had little detectable effect on hospitals' priorities.

Medical educators reinforced the priority accorded by physicians and therefore by hospitals to acute intervention and increasingly intensive care. The number of full-time clinicians in academic medicine grew by several orders of magnitude during the quarter century. The most rapid growth was in the surgical and diagnostic specialties and in cardiology and other subdisciplines of internal medicine. These specialists earned more income from clinical practice and often had larger research budgets than their colleagues in, for example, neurology, psychiatry, or pediatrics. The ability of invasive and diagnostic specialists to attract patients and research grants permitted them to claim more space and more capital to purchase equipment in teaching hospitals and medical schools. These clinicians and their similarly well-funded allies in the basic health sciences dominated the politics and thus the priorities of medical education throughout the quarter century. The ascendancy of academic clinicians and their allies had an enormous influence on health care. Reviewing this book in manuscript, Rosemary Stevens described that significance: "There was a closed acute system" in the United States after World War II, "fueled by the research ethos of the medical schools and their symbiotic relationship with leading hospitals."

The relatively low prestige of rehabilitation medicine among the specialties exemplifies the lower priority accorded to the disabling consequences of chronic illness and injury. Rehabilitation medicine emerged as a specialty during the war. It had been promoted in the press, especially as a result of the work of Dr. Howard Rusk with severely injured veterans. *The Best Years of Our Lives*, a film that won several Oscars in 1946, sentimentalized the achievements of rehabilitation medicine. Physical and rehabilitation medicine, the formal name of the new specialty, also appealed to many physicians and politicians because it was an alternative to social insurance for persons with permanent disabilities. To the leaders of organized medicine, any expansion of social insurance would increase the size of the constituency advocating national health insurance. Specialists in rehabilitation also protected medical territory and fees from encroachment by competing professionals, notably physical and occupational therapists, psychologists, and social workers. Mainly for these reasons, the AMA and its allies in the political center and on the right endorsed the expansion of the federal Vocational Rehabilitation Administration.[3]

The head of the Vocational Rehabilitation Administration for most of the quarter century after 1950 was Mary Switzer, a career civil servant who had helped plan the rapid growth of the National Institutes of Health in the postwar years. In 1954, anticipating the political success of a coalition supported by organized medicine, she told Alan Gregg of the Rockefeller Foundation that she now had "what we always wanted . . . the complete and unqualified commitment of the President and the national government to pursue rehabilitation as a major part of our national policy." But rehabilitation policy was never effectively linked to health policy, and rehabilitation medicine continued to have lower prestige among physicians than any other specialty except public health. Mary Switzer had not understood how strongly the most powerful people in the public and private sectors remained committed to the priorities of health policy that had been set at the beginning of the century.

Prominent members of President Eisenhower's cabinet articulated these older priorities. Marion B. Folsom, Switzer's superior as secretary of health, education and welfare, and George E. Humphrey, secretary of the treasury, had learned about the priorities of health policy as trustees of the hospitals that served, respectively, the University of Rochester and Western Reserve University. Together with Eisenhower's cardiologist, Paul Dudley White of Harvard and the Massachusetts General Hospital, Folsom and Humphrey urged the president to recommend that Congress increase the budget of the National Institutes of Health and authorize federal grants to help medical schools construct research facilities. Eisenhower did not seem to require much urging.

In numerous publications, the medical profession and its allies assimilated chronic illness to the priorities of a policy shaped in an earlier era. A representative pamphlet of the early 1950s, issued by a research organization financed by pharmaceutical companies, urged "apparently healthy persons" to visit "multi-test clinics," where they would receive a "screening test . . . for two or three or half a dozen, or a dozen diseases at a time." The first sentence of the pamphlet claimed that "chronic diseases constitute our modern day epidemics," citing an official of the U.S. Public Health Service as authority. According to the pamphlet, technologies for testing blood or X-raying organs could "point to the people who should . . . consult their physicians for diagnosis and treatment."[4]

The authors of this pamphlet and many similar exhortations about chronic disease communicated the same message that had been used to combat infection at the turn of the century—namely, that every person is at high risk of acquiring epidemic diseases caused by invisible microbes invading the body; therefore, every person should voluntarily submit to rigorous and impersonal laboratory procedures, so that physicians can identify the invaders and recommend action against them. The new message, in what would later be discarded as a simplistic analogy, substituted "degenerating organs" for "microbes."

A few contemporaries challenged this easy assimilation of chronic illness to older models of disease. Economist Eli Ginzberg, for instance, wrote in 1949 that many physicians "misconceived the potentialities of effectively controlling chronic illness largely because they have approached it in terms of a 'curative' bias which is easily explained by their training and experience."[5] The curative bias noted by Ginzberg and a few others was even visible in public health and welfare programs for the poor. New York City, for instance, established an Interdepartmental Health Council in 1953 to recommend action on the high priority assigned to chronic illness by national leaders of medicine and public health. In its investigation of the Department of Welfare's medical care programs, the council found that these programs were "primarily intended for the acutely ill" but were regularly providing "chronic care services" to 3,000 persons. Another 22,000 people in New York City, most of them with "diseases of the circulatory system," did not receive rehabilitative services but had recently become eligible for a new federal program of financial aid.[6]

According to council documents, the city's private and public hospitals were treating chronic diseases with methods devised in earlier times. A study of patients who were discharged over six months from a cross section of hospitals revealed that 24 percent had diagnoses of a chronic disease. Most of these persons were discharged after "short stays" (then defined as less than two weeks) without follow-up care for managing their conditions. Even Goldwater Hospital, established in the 1930s to conduct research on chronic disease and offer aggressive rehabilitative treatment of its consequences, had changed its mission. Half the beds at Goldwater were now used for custodial care that could have been rendered in nursing homes or in the patients' own homes. When King's County Hospital in Brooklyn proposed to the council that it establish a day care center for convalescing "aged hospital patients," an official of the health department declared that this was not "an appropriate use of hospital resources."

In 1951, in a book entitled *The Social System*, the distinguished sociologist Talcott Parsons assessed these conventional perceptions of illness. Parsons observed that most Americans and almost every health professional acted as if the only legitimate sickness occurred as a result of episodes of acute illness, whatever their cause and duration. Society classified these episodes, he wrote, as deviant behavior that violated norms and threatened the integrity of the social system. Other members of society then assigned the afflicted individuals to an appropriate "sick role." They were exempted from "normal social responsibilities," "taken care of," and obliged "to want to 'get well' " and to seek and "cooperate with" "technically competent" professional help. The social goal of managing sickness in society was to achieve the "balance of motivations to recover."[7]

Parsons believed that the sick role he described was a transient phenomenon in history. He wrote elsewhere in the same treatise that illness is "partly biologically and partly socially defined."

Moreover, he predicted that the "conceptual scheme of the biological science of the late nineteenth and early twentieth century
medicine" would not persist. He knew that acute infectious disease did not offer the only model for defining all disabling illness
and social responses to it. But he was studying a society in which
most people, and almost every physician, regarded illness as a
"disturbance in the 'normal' functioning of the total human individual," a disturbance from which substantial recovery was possible. Parsons knew very well that most illnesses were instead per-
sistent conditions that required continuous accommodation by
individuals and the institutions of society.[8] Persons with such conditions would regard improvements in their ability to function in
society as more attainable goals than recovery.

In the early 1960s, a few sociologists, notably Irving K. Zola,
revised Parsons's theory to take account of chronic disease and
disability.[9] These sociologists challenged descriptions of a sick role
that valued compliance with professional orders more highly than
independence and self-actualization. But most policy makers—
the people responsible for increasing the supply of research facilities, hospitals, and manpower to the health sector—continued to
assume that their role, like that of the Parsonian sick person, was
to cooperate with technically proficient professionals. A staff
member reported to President Eisenhower's director of the budget in 1960, for example, that

> through the unique device of advisory committees we are
> enabled to have essentially the same group of private citi-
> zens: 1) advise the Surgeon General on how much money he
> should request in his budget; 2) advise the Congress on how
> much money the Surgeon General should get; 3) apply for
> the grant money after it is made available; and, finally, 4)
> decide who should be awarded the grants. . . . [The] princi-
> pal advantage of the system is that it entirely eliminates
> confusion and uncertainty.[10]

Attempts to change the prevailing assumptions of health policy
were short-lived and usually unsuccessful. In the early months of
the Kennedy administration in 1961, for example, White House

officials who wanted to regain control of the NIH budget from Congress seemed to have something new in mind. The Eisenhower administration, wrote David Bell, Kennedy's budget director, had not recommended enough money for the NIH and had not recommended the right programs. Congress shared the erroneous view of the previous administration and a "large segment of the population that through 'crash programs' it might be possible to achieve major breakthroughs in the fight against our major killers, cancer and heart disease." Progress, Bell and his staff believed, would occur slowly and steadily if funding was adequate. The problems of chronic disease could not be solved by crash programs financed by a political system that embraced an expectant, Parsonian sick role.[11]

Like its predecessors and successors, however, the Kennedy administration returned—under the pressure of events—to the conventional assumptions that drove the politics of medical research. Kennedy recommended increasing the federal budget for research targeted at cancer, mental illness, and mental retardation; acquiesced in the established pattern of congressional domination of appropriations to NIH; and, over the opposition of his senior budget officials in 1963, established a presidential commission that assessed the diffusion of technology to treat acute episodes of heart disease, cancer, and stroke.[12]

During the negotiations that led to the passage of the Health Professions Education Assistance Act in 1962 and its subsequent extensions, moreover, the federal government and most of the provider interest groups assumed that much of the burden of illness was a result of a shortage of physicians and other health professionals—that is, a lack of people to diagnose and treat acute episodes. Over the next several years, subsidies to reduce this presumed shortage further increased the ratio of specialists to generalists in medical practice.

In 1967, however, budget officials in the Johnson administration devised incentives to induce medical schools to expand their enrollments and direct more of their graduates to specialties that managed the routine care of persons with chronic disabling illness in the community. These incentives, called capitation payments, became law in 1971 despite initial objections from lobbyists for the medical schools and high-ranking federal health officials. Medical school enrollments increased, but there were few recruits for what were now labeled the primary care specialties.[13]

Other initiatives of the Johnson administration reinforced prevailing priorities. The Comprehensive Health Planning (CHP) requirements enacted in 1966 became, in most states, a mechanism to ratify existing competitive relationships among powerful providers of high-technology health services, such as intensive care units and cobalt therapy machines. A few states, notably New York and Michigan, supplemented the CHP program with their own funds in order to regulate the supply of services for acute care. These states imposed mandatory approval of hospital capital expenditures (called certificates of need) instead of the voluntary agreements required by federal law. In New York, for instance, an alliance of state regulators, teaching hospital executives, and managers of Blue Cross plans had begun in 1964 to close inefficient small institutions and slow the rate at which community hospitals increased their beds and purchased expensive medical equipment.[14]

The Regional Medical Program (RMP) made even more explicit the prevailing assumptions about treating chronic disabling illness. This program was enacted in 1966 in response to a report prepared by the commission that President Kennedy had authorized in 1963. The assumption guiding RMP was that the management of heart disease, cancer, and stroke was inefficient largely because knowledge about useful interventions, developed in laboratories and teaching hospitals of medical schools, did not reach institutions and physicians in outlying communities. To solve this problem, RMP allocated federal funds to improve systems of diffusion. Two favorite methods were mobile diagnostic equipment and continuing medical education about new drugs and surgical techniques.

RMP is an extraordinarily clear example of both the paradox of health policy and the health policy compromise. Heart disease, cancer, and stroke are chronic illnesses that cause considerable disability and many deaths. Evidence was accumulating that their onset was preventable or at least postponable, mainly by changes in an individual's diet, exercise patterns, and consumption of tobacco and alcohol. Death was increasingly postponable when early symptoms of these diseases were diagnosed and treated. But RMP was conceived as a response to a public crisis, not to long-term trends in patterns of illness and methods of prevention and treatment. By focusing attention and funds on the acute phases of chronic disease, RMP reinforced the paradoxical mismatch between the allocation of resources and need. The program also reinforced the policy compromise by substituting an increase in the supply of services for diagnosis and acute care for increasing access to preventive services.

The story of RMP also illustrates how health policy accommodated to chronic diseases, even in a comparatively modest federal project targeted to academic medical centers. In some regions, staff paid by federal RMP grants decided to allocate more of their effort to improving patients' access to routine preventive and therapeutic care than to diffusing new technology. When the external evaluators chosen by officials of the Department of Health, Education and Welfare reported the positive results of this subversion of the program's goals, they were rewarded with a sole-source contract to perform a national evaluation of comprehensive health planning in the states and their component regions. These HEW officials, probably with tacit encouragement from the Bureau of the Budget, wanted—but not in public—to change rather than to reinforce existing systems for delivering health care.[15]

On the supply side of health affairs, in sum, policy makers, informed by experts, addressed the epidemiological and demographic pressures of the mid-twentieth century by modernizing the principles of health policy established at the turn of the century. They still assumed that most of the relevant knowledge aimed at improving health originated at the laboratory bench and that, on the basis of this knowledge, highly specialized physicians were devising interventions for acute phases of chronic disease. These interventions, which were initially tested in teaching hospitals, were then disseminated to less sophisticated institutions and professionals. The increasing prevalence of chronic disease merely raised the difficulties and therefore the costs of solving health problems; the solutions, however, were familiar and tested policies.

Chronic Disease and the Demand for Health Services

In the 1950s and 1960s, the leaders of the interest groups that struggled over how to pay for health services accorded priority to acute services, but they acknowledged the burden of chronic disabling disease by continuing the policy of gradual accommodation begun by their predecessors in the 1930s.

A competitive health insurance market had been created during the war by federal tax and labor policies that encouraged employers to substitute benefits for wage increases. By 1950, Blue Cross/Blue Shield plans and commercial insurers had approximately equal shares of this market. To the surprise of the executives of many commercial companies, health insurance had turned out to be profitable. Their profits and their growing market share were a result of their using the methods of liability insurance, especially experience rating. Insurance companies established premiums after determining the number of prior claims made by the persons insured in each group of employees. Because Blue Cross plans used social rather than liability insurance as their model, they determined the price for each subscriber by community rating—that is, prior claims by all the subscribers in a geographical area.[16] Blue Cross and commercial insurance companies also reimbursed providers, especially hospitals, in different ways. They both paid hospitals at a daily rate, up to a maximum number of days established for each calendar year in contracts with subscribers. Beginning in the mid-1950s, however, Blue Cross plans based the reimbursement for each day of care on an analysis of actual costs, whereas commercial firms paid charges or indemnities—negotiated prices for each unit of a covered service.

Experience rating gave the commercial companies a significant advantage in competing for the premiums of employee groups, which were composed predominantly of younger, healthier workers and their families. Under Blue Cross's community rating, healthier and generally younger subscribers and their employers subsidized health care for sicker and generally older workers, their dependents, and retired persons who continued to subscribe. Since there was no public policy to protect the Blues from competition with commercial insurance companies, and also no public subsidy for sicker people, Blue Cross coverage inevitably become more expensive than commercial insurance. For some years, many of the plans tried to compete with commercial insurance by increasing the size of their community-rated risk pools. By the late 1950s, however, most of the Blue plans had adopted experience rating for their larger corporate clients, their main source of subscribers. Community rating persisted, but only for employees of small businesses and for individual subscribers when states such as New York permitted Blue Cross to reimburse hospitals at a substantial discount below the charges paid by commercial insurers. This was not community rating on the original social insurance model, since many of the best risks were now covered by experience-rated plans. The subscribers who were now euphemistically called members of the "community" included a disproportionate number of employed persons and their dependents who had chronic diseases.

The commercial companies' method of reimbursing providers also gave them a competitive advantage. Whereas the Blues paid "service benefits" based on audited costs, the commercial companies paid negotiated charges or indemnities. This method of payment gave them more control over their own costs than the Blues had. As a result, they could market their policies at lower prices by requiring beneficiaries to share more of the risk through deductibles and copayments. Commercial health insurance could then be marketed on the same profitable basis as coverage for damage to property.

To actuaries, the incidence and the costs of disease and disability in any group are predictable risks. The practical problem for insurance companies is to remain profitable while meeting their customers' demand for protection from the risk of illness that had, in the new phrase of the time, "catastrophic costs." Beginning in 1950, insurance companies tried to solve this problem by offering major medical insurance. These policies paid for hospital and medical treatment of all diseases, with deductibles and coinsurance, up to a large dollar limit. By 1955, two and a half million people and their employers had purchased major medical insurance. As a result, about 1 percent of Americans with health insurance had extensive coverage; by 1961, the number had grown to 6 percent.

Major medical insurance, like experience rating, was a threat to Blue Cross and Blue Shield plans. Some plans offered their own versions of major medical coverage. Others—for instance, the plan in New York City, the largest in the country—insisted until the late 1960s that service benefits without coinsurance or deductibles cost less and provided more coverage for the average family than the indemnities of major medical insurance. In 1953, Rufus Rorem, still working for the National Blue Cross Commission, insisted that "coverage for chronic illness" was one of seven standards for measuring the comparative adequacy of the commercial plans that were competing with Blue Cross.

The Blues devised new strategies to compete with major medical insurance for customers who feared the costs of managing chronic disabling illness. Most of the plans subsidized benefits for elderly subscribers with the payments of younger and healthier subscribers in their community-rated risk pools. In the 1960s, during the debate about health insurance for the elderly, a number of plans publicly identified the amount of this subsidy. Almost all the plans added benefits to meet competition from commercial insurers. Many plans paid hospital benefits for up to 120 days. A number of plans extended eligibility for service benefits to hospitals that offered care mainly to persons who had specified chronic diseases. Still others covered the costs of nursing home stays and home health care following periods of hospitalization.

In 1954 and 1955, the Eisenhower administration proposed to subsidize the pooling of the risks of the catastrophic costs of illness that were underwritten by voluntary insurance. Such reinsurance insulates insurance companies, at a price, from large losses caused by policyholders with the highest risks. The Eisenhower administration's proposal, which was supported by the Blue Cross and Blue Shield plans, would have reduced the competitive advantage of experience-rated plans. It failed in Congress because of opposition from commercial insurance companies; fiscal conservatives; organized medicine and its allies, who feared setting a precedent for federal intervention; and liberals, who thought it did not go far enough.[17]

An exasperated President Eisenhower would not be the last national leader to discover that ideology and interests, rather than logic, drive policy to meet the demand for health care. He could not understand, he told the Republican leader of the Senate, the intensity of opposition to a plan that "would have shown the people how we could improve their health and stay out of socialized medicine."[18]

Pressure increased during the 1950s for the federal and state governments to participate in financing health care for persons with chronic disabling illness. In the 1940s, several states had created modest programs of health care linked to disability. In 1950, in response to growing state costs for medical care to the poor, especially the aged poor, the federal government authorized grants to the states to pay vendors of medical services to the needy aged and persons who were permanently and totally disabled. By the end of the decade, persons in every category of public welfare were eligible for federal subsidies of payments by the states.[19]

The amendments to the Social Security Act in 1956—which created Social Security Disability Insurance (SSDI), initially only for persons over the age of fifty—had considerable significance for health policy. The leading interest groups in health affairs recognized that a social insurance program that provided incomes for people with disabilities could become a model for an analogous program to provide health services to the same people, to the elderly, or even to everyone. The officials who managed disability insurance had considerably more discretion than their counterparts who were responsible for the old-age pensions enacted in the Social Security Act of 1935. Ascertaining eligibility for an old-age retirement program required only inspection of proof of age and of evidence that premiums had been paid for a minimum period of time. A disability program required policy to define when particular impairments caused sufficient disability to merit initial and continuing payment and how and by whom these determinations would be made. Disability programs generated considerable litigation, as workers' compensation had demonstrated.

The debate about federal disability insurance in 1956 was acrimonious, as it had been on several earlier occasions. The Eisenhower administration opposed SSDI partly on fiscal grounds but also in deference to the AMA and commercial insurance companies. Organized labor and senior career civil servants in the Social Security Administration were its major supporters. After the House of Representatives passed the bill, it was introduced in the Senate as a floor amendment, in order to avoid powerful opponents on the Finance Committee. There it passed by two votes, but the White House decided against a veto. Almost immediately, some members of Congress began to say that the next step should be national health insurance, beginning with medical care for the elderly.

The creation of SSDI was one among many political events that made possible the passage of Medicare in 1965. As a rich literature describes, these events include the election of an increasing number of liberals to Congress, and especially to the Senate, beginning in 1958; the successful effort by the American Association of Retired Persons and other organizations to mobilize elderly people to support social insurance for health care; the influence of public opinion—which strongly favored expanding Social Security—on political decisions at the beginning of the Kennedy administration; the skillful political work of Wilbur Cohen and other government social policy professionals; the landslide electoral victory of Lyndon Johnson in 1964 and the strong liberal majorities in the 89th Congress; and the legislative ingenuity of Congressman Wilbur Mills and other leaders in the final months before passage.[20]

Most accounts of these events, however, ignore the consensus in 1965 that Medicare should not directly address the growing burden of chronic disabling illness. This consensus extended beyond Medicare to include Medicaid, the federal-state program of means-tested medical, hospital, and long-term care that was passed at the same time. During the negotiations preceding the passage of Medicare and Medicaid, officials of the Johnson administration insisted that both programs would give priority to care during acute episodes of illness. The secretary of health, education and welfare, for example, said in testimony to Congress that Medicare was not a program to pay the costs of managing chronic illness in short-stay hospitals. Other officials claimed to be horrified when Russell Long, chairman of the Senate Finance Committee, proposed amendments to Medicare to create a "catastrophic or long-term illness system." This insistence that Medicare and Medicaid were programs to pay for treatment of acute conditions was a political tactic. Administration strategists feared that they would lose supporters in Congress, especially in the House Ways and Means Committee, if the program appeared to be uncontrollably expensive.

Medicare, in fact, was the most extensive program for the care of chronic illness that had ever been proposed in the United States, either by government or by nonprofit or commercial insurers. It covered considerably more extended care than any contemporary insurance plan: up to sixty days of nursing home service and 240 days of home health care in a calendar year. Administration officials told Congress, with more confidence than evidence, that the costs of this care could be controlled because it would be permitted only after patients were discharged from hospitals following acute episodes of precisely diagnosable disease. To administration officials and congressional leaders, this was a familiar and comfortable argument. For almost two decades, decision makers had been accommodating the supply of health services, as well as the methods of financing them, to the burden of chronic illness. In 1965, this burden was again addressed by policies that officially gave priority to treating acute episodes of illness. Contrary to official statements, however, Medicare, and to an even greater extent Medicaid, enormously increased the resources allocated to the supply and financing of services for chronic disabling illness.

This pattern of accommodation reflected the compromise

reached by divergent interest groups: a mixed system of voluntary and social insurance and means-tested benefits. A social insurance system that covered and taxed everyone could conceivably have paid the high cost of explicitly addressing chronic disease. However, the current system—in which commercial and nonprofit plans still competed on both price and coverage—was designed to finance care for discrete episodes of acute illness rather than care that extended over indeterminate periods of time.

A 1972 amendment to the enabling legislation for Medicare did insure treatment for one chronic illness, kidney disease. The politics that preceded this amendment began more than a decade earlier, in response to advances in dialysis and techniques for surgical transplantation. Most voluntary health insurance did not cover these expensive new interventions. Moreover, there were never enough donated organs and, at the beginning, too few dialysis machines to meet demand. As a result, physicians were making explicit decisions to ration treatment, using criteria they derived from their moral and social values as well as from pathophysiology. Physicians, patients, and the media criticized such allocative decision making.

In 1966, the federal Bureau of the Budget (BoB) appointed, secretly, a committee of nongovernmental experts chaired by Carl W. Gottschalk, M.D., to assess the issue. Consistent with the health policy compromise, BoB officials assumed that medical research created imperatives for financing that should be accepted without question. "This endeavor settled in the Bureau because the tremendous costs involved appeared to be more overriding than scientific or technological implications," a BoB official told his chief.[21] The Gottschalk Committee, by now identified in public, recommended in 1967 that the benefits of dialysis and transplantation exceeded the costs and that it was in the public interest to pay for them.

In 1972, Congress, influenced by interest groups rather than by this expert report, enacted what appeared, but only superficially, to be an amendment that contradicted the health policy compromise. Under the new law, persons who had what was now called end-state renal disease (ESRD) were entitled to full coverage for dialysis and transplantation (but not immunosuppressive drugs) under Medicare. The ESRD program used the premiums of social insurance (every working person's Social Security tax) to spread the cost of reasonably effective treatment for the acute, life-threatening manifestations of a chronic degenerative disease. But the program did not contradict the terms of the policy compromise, since it narrowly limited its benefits to the final acute stage of the disease and anticipated much lower expenditures than actually occurred. A BoB assessment had complained that the Gottschalk Committee's report had this deficiency. More important, Wilbur Mills, powerful chairman of the House Committee on Ways and Means, insisted that the purpose of the bill in 1972 was to provide "necessary life-saving care and treatment."[22] The phrase *end-stage renal disease* was essentially invented to fit the assumptions of Medicare and the health policy compromise, not the pathophysiology of nephritis.

Thus, the ESRD program did not foreshadow universal coverage or even reveal a new sensitivity to the tough policy issues raised by chronic disease. The program merely provided additional evidence that, when treatment is available for acute conditions, Americans find it repugnant to ration care to particular individuals on the basis of their character, their social worth, or their wealth.

On the other hand, Medicaid, the means-tested welfare program, actually offered more extensive coverage for chronic disabling illness than either Medicare or private insurance. The explicit purpose of Medicaid was to provide basic medical services for recipients of categorical welfare benefits and for people whom each state would define as medically needy. Within a few years, however, Medicaid was providing considerable long-term care, in institutions and at home, for persons of all ages with chronic disabling conditions. In the early 1970s, the first historians of Medicaid, Rosemary and Robert Stevens, observed with some surprise that the program "positively encouraged elderly persons to go to nursing homes after a period in hospital."

This change in the purpose and very soon the cost of Medicaid was a result of its origin as welfare rather than health policy.

Eligibility and benefit levels for public welfare have traditionally been decided on the basis of moral and political rather than medical criteria. Illness and injury have been relatively uncontroversial causes of eligibility for welfare, because many sick or disabled people are demonstrably unable to work. During periods of relative prosperity and the ascendancy of political coalitions that include liberals, the benefits of public welfare programs have usually become increasingly generous. In the 1960s, prosperity and politics combined to enact Medicaid, a program that, following the tradition of public welfare, created an entitlement to long-term care that was virtually open-ended for persons who were eligible for it.

The health policy compromise, except for Medicaid, was driven mainly by medical criteria—that is, by the assumptions about science, technology, and disease that had been the basis of health policy since the turn of the century. The compromise was a set of agreements about how to supply and finance services to eliminate the causes and treat the acute symptoms of diagnosable disease. Medicaid, which was welfare rather than health policy, was, as a political scientist has described it, "plastic," shaped by clients' needs as they were defined by the morality and politics of the time.[23] Other health policy responded to need only indirectly. On the supply side, policy sought to advance and diffuse medical science. Policy to meet the demand for care sought, however tortuously, to calculate and finance treatment for the risks of pathological events whose consequences could be precisely calculated.

The Uniqueness of United States Health Policy

Almost alone among industrial nations, the United States does not ensure access to health services to everyone through a program paid for by public or private funds or some combination of them. We offer access to health services mainly on the basis of age, income, and employment. How much access people with jobs have is mainly a result of the size of their employer's work force and the extent to which they benefit from collective bargaining. The benefits we provide through both voluntary and social insurance disadvantage persons who require extensive and expensive care over long periods of time. Many persons of working age and their dependents have no coverage for long-term care for severely disabling illness or injury.

There are a number of plausible explanations for our unique health financing policy.[24] Some explanations emphasize American values and characteristics. Specifically, according to these explanations, our emphasis on individualism and minimal government has made it difficult to build effective coalitions to promote social policy. In addition, our optimism about material progress and human perfectibility has sustained policies directed at solving social and health problems by science and technology; our optimism also is responsible for the widespread belief that individual prosperity and good health can substitute for a social policy aimed at reducing the costs of health services to individuals.

Other explanations emphasize the power of particular interest groups, such as physicians and other producer groups, in the formation of health policy. According to the proponents of these explanations, these groups have attained power in our political system because, unlike Western European countries, we do not have powerful labor unions or a political party that relies primarily on working-class votes (or, indeed, many people who describe themselves as working class). In a country that makes new policy mainly in response to crises, moreover, we have not had a crisis in health service that stimulated more than incremental changes in policy. In addition, because of the enormous power of provider groups, health services have become a bigger business in the United States than in other countries, so that more people (in 1993, almost 10 percent of the nation's work force) have a stake in maintaining existing policies.

In comparison with other industrial countries, the United States, throughout the twentieth century, has had a limited sense of collective responsibility for illness and its consequences in disability and suffering. This is a troubling claim to make about a country whose citizens and leaders take pride in their generosity to people in need. I illustrate it by comparison with the United Kingdom.[25]

When I began to study the history of policy for chronic illness and disability in Britain, I was struck by the similarity in what was important to provider interest groups, the media, and various decision makers in both countries; that is, all these groups gave priority to acute services. At the inception of the National Health Service (NHS), British leaders, political as well as medical, had about the same view of the relative priority of services for acute and chronic phases of disease as the health specialists in the Democratic or Republican parties, or for that matter the AFL-CIO and the National Association of Manufacturers, in the United States. In 1945, when the British Ministry of Health was planning the NHS, Sir Wilson Jameson, the chief medical officer, wrote in his annual report on the nation's health that "doctors both in this country and the United States have been taking an interest in the problems of care" for aged and chronically sick persons. Yet, he continued, the "care of the chronic sick has tended [in Britain as in the United States] to be regarded as uninteresting, uninspiring and depressing." In the same report, Sir Wilson published, but did not explicate, tables that showed chronic disease accounting for about five times more British deaths than war-related injuries had between 1940 and 1945. In Sir Wilson's view, the task of establishing the National Health Service distracted the ministry from its concerns about chronic illness.[26]

There are other similarities in the priorities of policy in Britain and the United States. In both countries, physicians who specialize in managing chronic disabling disease have complained about being accorded low priority. Geriatric medicine, for instance, which was established as a specialty in Britain in the 1930s, has had low prestige, just as rehabilitation medicine and, later, geriatrics have had in the United States. In both countries, many so-called chronics—persons with disabling illness—have been stigmatized because they did not act out socially approved sick roles, which were defined by acute episodes of illness. Moreover, in both Britain and the United States, charitable organizations promoting policy on behalf of particular diseases or disabling conditions often helped to fragment concern about chronic illness in general. As Raymond Illisley, a British social scientist long active in health affairs, told me, "I cannot think of anybody in this country who is interested in chronic disease, just in *particular* chronic diseases."[27]

There are also similarities between the policies of the two countries, especially research policy. The Medical Research Council of Great Britain began to accord explicit priority to research on chronic diseases in the 1930s, at about the same time that leading American medical scientists first advocated a shift in policy. Significant clinical research on chronic diseases—notably heart disease, cancer, and rheumatoid arthritis—was carried out, sometimes collaboratively, in both countries.[28] There are even unexpected similarities in policy for financing health services. In both countries, the health sector is a large employer, especially in the hospital sector. British policy analyst Rudolf Klein has noted that doctors and other employees of the National Health Service have exploited periodic crises about the availability of acute health services in order to increase public appropriations.[29] Similarly, the media in the United States have since 1960 routinely declared access to acute services to be in crisis. In both countries, experts and commissions have since the 1930s regularly deplored the availability and quality of services for people with chronic illness.

Nevertheless, health policy in the two countries affects persons with chronically disabling disease and injury very differently. Policy in Britain has, in general, taken more account of populations, whereas policy in the United States has more frequently been driven by concern about particular diseases. In the 1960s, for example, the National Health Service introduced a new planning concept, the "young chronic sick" (people from adolescence to late middle age), which remains unknown in the United States.[30] By the mid-1970s, in response to criticism that data about populations were not being considered when resources were allocated, Britain began to adjust its health policy. As part of the reforms in the National Health Service of the 1990s, some purchasing authorities are beginning to refine and restructure care in the community on the basis of evidence derived from population studies.

In 1993, the government accepted recommendations made first by a foundation-sponsored inquiry and then by an official commission to transfer resources in London from hospitals to care in the community. If these recommendations are actually carried out over the next decade, they will result in more extensive redistribution of effort from acute care to the management of chronic illness than has yet occurred in any jurisdiction.[31]

The United Kingdom has also had relatively more effective policy than the United States for paying the costs of long-term care and managing the consequences of chronic illness. The central concept of the NHS is that the costs of everyone's illnesses are spread over every taxpayer. Britain adjusted more easily to the increasing demand for services as a result of the burden of chronic illness because, like most industrial countries, it spread risk and the payment of cost over the largest conceivable group.

The United Kingdom is also relatively more effective than the United States in providing care in the community, especially for severely ill children and the frail elderly. This claim is controversial. British advocates of improvements in their system who are unfamiliar with health care in the United States often insist that ours could not conceivably be worse than theirs. American advocates for improved services for persons with disabling motor and sensory conditions and mental retardation often cite reports of limited access to similar services in the United Kingdom. Americans with severely disabling conditions who have financial resources and advocates—people with cerebral palsy, the deaf, and the blind, for example—have probably been better served than their counterparts in Britain. On the other hand, the average person with a chronic illness or disabling condition has probably had better access to health and social services in the United Kingdom.[32]

Contrary to conventional opinion, Americans' belief in a strong private sector has not been the fundamental reason for differences between our health policy and that of other countries. In every industrial country, major areas of health policy have remained the responsibility of the private sector, and health policy has been continuously influenced by well-organized private sector interest groups. Moreover, as many observers have pointed out, physicians in the United States are much more heavily regulated by the state and by insurers than their counterparts are in Europe.

Britain and other industrial countries devised different health policies than the United States primarily because they achieved a workable consensus about the value of sharing responsibility for health and well-being. Policy makers in these countries, like those in the United States, believed they were according the highest priority to acute care; but they established policies that spread the costs of all illnesses over everyone who could pay them, and they made everyone eligible for care. Each case of severe chronic disabling illness or injury was a human, not a financial, catastrophe. In the aggregate, therefore, chronic illness has been a smaller relative burden on European health plans than on most employee insurance groups in the United States. Our health policy has been unable to defy the statistical law of large numbers.

The United States, in sum, has unevenly applied the concept of shared responsibility for health and well-being to the financing of personal health services. Americans applied the concept most generously in Medicaid, a program that was vulnerable to changes in morality and politics—vulnerable, to be more precise, to racism, recession, and the breakdown of the New Deal coalition. They had applied it in a more limited way in Medicare, but only to the elderly and, after 1972, also to persons receiving Social Security Disability Insurance and those with end-stage renal disease. Moreover, Medicare, which was conceived as an insurance and not a general welfare program, tied benefits for long-term care to episodes of acute illness. The health policy compromise in the United States was more fragile, more vulnerable to other changes in politics and the economy, than its analogues elsewhere.

4

Health Policy in Disarray, 1975-1993

The compromise on health policy devised in the third quarter of the century continued into the 1990s despite widespread dissatisfaction with it. This dissatisfaction was a legacy of the paradox of resource allocation established early in the century. Policy still stimulated both an increasing supply of services for acute intervention and a rising demand for them. At the same time, more people needed help to prevent, postpone, and manage the disabling consequences of chronic illnesses. As a result of the persistence of both the paradox and the compromise, the costs of health care continued to increase; at the same time, many people had inadequate access to routine care for chronic illness, and many others had to rely on public charity for acute medical and hospital services.

An expert who read this chapter in manuscript form suggested that it might be titled "The Great Deceit." The American people, after accepting almost a century of propaganda that they had the best health system in the world, began in the past two decades to discover that it was only the world's most expensive. That is too strong a judgment for me; but it could be made about much of the evidence that follows.

Since the 1970s, for the first time in this century, there has been public debate involving leaders of business, philanthropy, and government about who should have what authority in health affairs, under what rules, and judged by what criteria of success and failure. The priorities and governance of health affairs had not been so open to challenge since the turn of the century, when a recently organized coalition transformed the purposes and institutions of health care. Most of the leaders of that coalition were academic physicians. They were supported by business leaders, philanthropists, and officials of state and local government.

The priorities of health policy established at the beginning of the century persisted because they were sustained by persuasive ideas and supported by effective interest groups. Even when, in the early twentieth century, they were confronted with a growing incidence and prevalence of chronic disabling illness, policy makers retained their existing priorities for policy. Most of them assumed that chronic disabling illness could eventually be prevented and treated without any changes in their assumptions about the best ways to supply and finance health services. During the third quarter of the century, policy makers negotiated a compromise to supply and pay for health services for most Americans. This compromise ensured that knowledge about chronic disabling illness and the supply of professionals and facilities to treat it would increase. It also ensured continuing anxiety about the costs and adequacy of health services.

The health policy compromise has been this country's variation on the international concept of the welfare state. Like people in other industrial countries, American taxpayers share some of the responsibility for the risks of illness and death. But we have been unwilling to share all the predictable risks, especially the risks of chronic disabling illness. Moreover, we do not share the risks of sickness or disability as equitably as most other Western countries do.

Adjusting the Compromise

The health policy compromise was in disarray by the early 1980s. The politics that created the compromise had made it expensive.

Public and private policy to supply health services had stimulated rapid growth in spending for research, hospitals, pharmaceuticals, equipment, and the education of professionals. Government and the insurance industry paid the bills for care in ways that encouraged physicians to prescribe services, especially procedures, and also encouraged patients to use these services.

The compromise also caused considerable anxiety. Private employers were anxious because the rising costs of health care for their employees and retirees reduced corporate profits; public officials, because the costs increased pressure on them to raise taxes, reduce benefits, or eliminate beneficiaries. People without any insurance, as well as those whose insurance did not cover their illness or disability or that of their dependents, worried about paying for care, especially as they became older and more vulnerable to chronic disabling illness. People covered by Medicare worried about the rising costs of treating catastrophic illnesses and of long-term care at home or in nursing homes. Recipients of Medicaid worried about losing their eligibility because either their personal economic situation improved or that of their state became worse.

Interest groups continuously either sought or fought against adjustments in the compromise that were intended to address rising cost and the anxiety it caused. Advocates of more extensive reforms than adjustments, especially those who looked to other industrial countries for models, were usually ignored in the negotiations among contending interest groups and public officials. These negotiations have created a great deal of new policy since the 1970s:

Federal and state restraints on hospital spending for construction and equipment.

Federal legislation offering incentives to increase the number of health maintenance organizations and enrollment in them.

The negotiation by employers and insurance plans of significant discounts from hospitals and physicians.

Payments to hospitals under Medicare for episodes of illness rather than days of service.

The beginning of redistribution of some medical fees paid
   by Medicare from invasive to primary care specialists.
More intrusive review, by insurers and their agents, of the
   services ordered by physicians.
Increases in Medicaid eligibility and benefits for children
   and their mothers.
State Medicaid initiatives to transfer resources from
   hospitals to care by physicians and agencies in
   communities.
State initiatives to provide insurance coverage for persons
   who have low incomes or high risks or who work in
   small firms.

Almost all these adjustments to the compromise addressed the
cost and availability of acute care. There were a few exceptions:
a handful of demonstration projects under Medicare that linked
long-term to acute care; incentives to the states under Medicaid
to expand home and community-based care for persons with
chronic disabling illness; a few clinical preventive services added
by Congress to Medicare; and a few preventive measures, most
frequently smoking cessation, covered by a small number of voluntary health insurance plans. The most significant increase in
preventive services occurred in Medicaid benefits for children and
pregnant women.

Acute care received priority in these adjustments for several
reasons. The most obvious reason was the pressure of immediate
events. The costs of acute care were rising. What people without
any health insurance wanted most urgently was medical and hospital care for acute conditions. The most significant advocacy for
policy to provide more care for persons with chronic disabling
illness came from organizations representing the elderly. But
these organizations' demands could usually be deflected by political leaders because older Americans had already, as a group, been
transformed from penury to relative affluence by Social Security
and Medicare.

Advocates of a higher priority for preventive services were even
easier to deflect. Most of the people who made or influenced
health policy were ambivalent about prevention. On the one hand,

as concerned citizens, they recognized that Americans might be able to prevent or postpone the onset of particular chronic diseases by modifying their behavior, especially their diets, exercise habits, and use of alcohol and tobacco. On the other hand, many of them were reluctant to add preventive measures, especially those that required counseling and education, to lists of reimbursed health services or to increase the resources of public health agencies. In part, this resistance was a result of prudent financial management: do not spend money for prevention now or next year when it is not at all clear whether, or when, or in whose budget savings will occur.[1]

The resistance to prevention among decision makers in the private and public sectors has a long history. From the 1890s to the 1980s, experts and advocates in health affairs promised that increasing the supply of facilities, professionals, and research would lead first to more successful and available technology for diagnosis and treatment and then to better health for Americans. Preventive services that could be delivered by injections or in tablet form fulfilled this promise. Prevention that required people to change their behavior was, however, outside the conditions of the promise. The promise of better health through procedures administered by professionals was central to policy to support medical education, to define health insurance benefits, and to establish priorities for research. Changing these policies would be difficult, perhaps impossible.

Most important, acute care was accorded priority in adjusting the compromise because most decision makers in government and the private sector, always describing themselves as realists, believed that they had no alternative. More services for persons with chronic disabling illness might, in theory, be desirable. But adding new priorities to health policy had always increased costs. Moreover, in the day-to-day political work of adjusting the compromise, any effort to shift priority from acute care without also increasing overall expenditures provoked vivid and potentially dangerous antagonism. Nobody who is accountable to voters or boards of directors or dues-paying members likes to be accused of, for example, rationing, infanticide, murder, or even of tossing people out of lifeboats, blaming victims, or playing God. It is much safer to deny these accusations and remain focused on providing, funding, insuring, teaching about, or doing research on better medical and hospital care for acute conditions.

The politics of health affairs were, however, slowly changing. These changes had two immediate causes. First, a conservative political resurgence that began in the 1960s transformed both major political parties and the institutions of government at every level. Second, leaders in American society, especially business executives, were no longer willing to permit members of the medical profession to make autonomous decisions about patient care and to guide the priorities of health policy.

The Center-Right Coalition and Health Policy

As a result of a conservative resurgence that began in the 1960s, a new coalition took control of the legislative, executive, and judicial branches of the federal government. A center-right array of political alliances became for more than a decade the norm of national politics, changing the trend of our social policy. The extent of that change should not be exaggerated. On the one hand, there has been considerable continuity in social policy under the center-right coalition. The Social Security system remains intact. Categorical public welfare programs have been diminished or reoriented but not abolished. Much of what has been called "America's misunderstood welfare state" retains effective political support.[2] On the other hand, the assumptions that many people made about what government should do, especially at the federal level, have been transformed. As a result, the terms of political debate have changed considerably.

From the 1930s to the early 1970s—more precisely, from the election of Franklin D. Roosevelt to the unraveling of Richard M. Nixon's presidency—most Americans on the winning side of federal and state politics had assumed that increasing centralization of authority in a strong federal government and in large private institutions was inevitable. A consensus about centralization dominated national politics during this period. The consensus was that important decisions about the economy and the welfare of society should be made by leaders of Congress and the executive branch and by the leaders of major nongovernment institutions (corporations and nonprofit organizations, professional associations, and industrial labor unions). An influential analysis published in the early 1980s summarized this theme in the title "Dwight D. Eisenhower and the Corporate Commonwealth."[3]

For four decades, most voters and leaders in the public and private sectors believed that the centralizing coalition would give Americans what they wanted: high employment rates and rising real wages; reasonably equal opportunity for members of all social groups to obtain jobs and start businesses; protection against Communists abroad and criminals at home; low interest rates and affordable down payments on home mortgages; faster and safer roads and highways; health care for everyone at reasonable prices; income security for the elderly, persons with severe disability, and people without work through no fault of their own; and more access to higher education.

The coalition that accepted the inevitability of centralization varied in political strength during its ascendancy; it was weakest from 1946 to 1948 and from 1953 to 1956, strongest in 1934–37 and 1964–66. Throughout its ascendancy, the coalition looked to liberals to supply most of its initiatives in social policy. The liberals who dominated social policy tried to Americanize aspects of the Western European and Canadian welfare state. The most prominent of these social policy experts from the 1930s to the 1980s was Wilbur Cohen.[4]

Many people had economic and social goals that were similar to those of the centralizing alliance, but they deplored the methods the coalition used to achieve these goals, especially in social policy. These people called themselves conservatives, classical liberals, libertarians, states' rights advocates, and, more recently, neoconservatives and neoliberals. They distrusted solutions to social and economic problems that required government action, especially action by the federal government. Instead, they preferred to achieve economic and social goals by using the competitive discipline of a market economy. For most conservatives, that economy would be healthiest if it encouraged competition among many small and medium-sized firms. Government should not encourage or protect bigness in either business or labor, and should interfere as little as possible in the production and distribution of goods and services.[5]

Many conservatives had a social policy agenda. In their view, poverty and its consequences were mainly the result of failure to use the market properly as an instrument to create and distribute wealth. Market failure worsened the character flaws of many poor people. Flawed character was reinforced by generous public welfare policies that, for example, did not exchange benefits for work and therefore discouraged people from helping themselves. As remedies for the failure to use market discipline, conservatives advocated incentives to poor people to seek employment, vouchers to purchase education and rehabilitation services from private or public vendors, and tax policies that encouraged savings and investment. In addition, a "safety net" of social welfare programs should be available for people who experienced personal catastrophes and for those too young, old, or disabled to participate in the market.

These conservatives regarded health care as a commodity, like any other commodity in the marketplace. Some economists, notably Milton Friedman, had been asserting since the 1940s that health services should not have privileged status as public or collective goods. Defining health services as special because of the uncertainty inherent in the physician-patient relationship, they said, protected from the market the people who produced services, thereby creating monopolistic power and making it difficult to restrain rising costs.[6] Restoring health services to the discipline of the market would be the best way to control escalating costs. The market also offered a way to avoid the limitations of voluntary health insurance if conservatives could persuade their allies in the political center to repeal policies that offered incentives to inefficiency and rising costs. The most important of these policies were the exclusion from taxable income of the value of benefits linked to employment and state mandates that required insurers to cover particular services.

Many conservatives also had what they euphemistically called a social agenda. Items on this agenda that involved sexuality, family planning, and abortion gave them additional justification for opposing the health policies they associated with the welfare state.

The politics of the center-right coalition were complicated. Many of its supporters disagreed with some aspects of the social policy or social agendas of their allies. Similarly, many supporters of the center-left centralizing coalition that had been dominant for so long were opposed to abortion on demand or to liberal civil rights policies or objected to generous health and welfare benefits. Moreover, interest groups with stakes in health policy—including employers, unions, insurers, physicians, and pharmaceutical companies—contributed to the election campaigns of candidates across the political spectrum. Nevertheless, a growing number of voters were in favor of changing fundamental assumptions about what should and could be done in national politics. The center-right coalition elected a president in 1980 who promised lower marginal rates for federal income tax and reduced domestic spending. In the next few years, center-right distrust of federal authority became operational in the continuing deregulation of industries, the delegation of human service programs to the states, and sizable reductions in federal contributions to these programs.

For most of the 1980s, however, the center-right coalition appeared to sustain the health policy compromise negotiated in the 1950s and 1960s, despite the eagerness of its most conservative members for reform. A plausible argument could be made that the center-right was responsible for only one major change in health politics between the mid-1970s and the early 1990s: it discouraged congressional liberals from engaging in the annual ritual of introducing bills that would provide comprehensive national health insurance and a single government payer.

During the 1980s, moreover, the federal government actually strengthened aspects of the compromise. The NIH budget continued to grow. The Reagan administration initially promoted diagnosis related groups (DRGs) in 1982 as a way to control hospital costs using market-oriented incentives. Each DRG would be a price for an episode of hospitalization. Efficient hospitals would make money; others would break even or lose. But, in practice, DRGs proved to be complicated, centralized regulation of institutional behavior. Medicare costs and central control also grew when it began to pay for hospice care and increased benefits for home health care. Another change in Medicare, the short-lived program passed in 1989 to pay the costs of catastrophic illness by taxing the more affluent recipients of Social Security, signaled that some members of the center-right coalition supported incremental increases in the benefits provided under the compromise. Similarly, the center-right leadership of Congress agreed to expand Medicaid coverage for women and children and to permit workers who were laid off to continue their health benefits for eighteen months. The only reversal in health policy as a result of the turn to the right seemed to be the elimination of federal support for health planning in the states.

This evidence that most of the compromise persisted was only part of the story, however. As conservatives repeatedly warned, events in Washington were never entirely representative of what was happening in the country. Beginning in the mid-1970s, the people who paid most of the costs of care—business firms, insurers, and state government officials—challenged fundamental assumptions of health policy.

The Decline of Medical Authority

The authority accorded to physicians began to decline in the 1970s. According to John Burnham and other historians, a "Golden Age" of medicine began in the 1920s and lasted until the late 1960s.[7] During that period, the values and preferences of physicians determined what services were available and how health care was organized. As a result, physicians became more highly esteemed and more handsomely paid than any other occupational group. First the press and then radio, the movies, and television idealized physicians and their work. Demand for admission to medical schools grew to its highest level in the 1960s and early 1970s. Government and philanthropic subsidies for medical research increased. Medicare and Medicaid fueled another spurt in physicians' incomes; what had been doctors' charity now became their receipts. As a result of the growth in Medicare and Medicaid payments to teaching hospitals and their medical staffs, academic physicians, for the first time, demanded and soon received parity in pay and benefits with specialists in community practice.

The Golden Age of medical dominance of health policy ended because of three sets of events. One was worry about the performance of the American economy. A second was behavior by physicians and other suppliers of health services that justified the conservative economists' description of them as producers and sellers of commodities. The third was that many people began to doubt that advancing medical knowledge about diagnosis and treatment would be the major cause of longer life and better health. These events transformed the politics of health affairs. Most important, for the first time since the 1890s, leading business executives questioned, even criticized, the priorities for health policy urged on them by leaders of the medical profession.

The transformation remains incomplete. Physicians retain extraordinary power and trust and, in return, command substantial rewards. They continue to write the orders and prescribe the tests, drugs, and treatments that drive most expenditures for patient care. Many physicians still influence business leaders' views about health policy. Most of the business executives who serve as trustees of hospitals, for example, continue to endorse physicians' priorities; but many of these trustees are asking more searching questions than they did in the past.

Business and Medicine: The End of the Special Relationship

Physicians and business executives devised a special relationship beginning in the 1890s. Business executives assumed that most physicians always tried to act in the best interests of their patients; therefore, business groups usually adopted the views of organized medicine about health policy. In return, most physicians and their organizations supported business leaders' positions on local, state, and national policy. Family and social ties reinforced the special relationship; so did the presentation of physicians as selfless heroes in novels, the movies, and television.[8]

The special relationship has gradually ended and is being replaced by wariness and even antagonism. Many physicians in fee-for-service practice snarl or wince at the euphemisms "utilization review" and "managed care," because it is *their* decisions about what to prescribe and how to treat that are being reviewed and, often, managed. The major support for these restraints on the practice of medicine comes from business—either directly, for the many large firms that self-insure, or from insurance companies and Blue Cross plans eager to attract and retain corporate customers in a highly competitive market.

Although many business executives still have warm relationships with their personal physicians and with relatives and friends in the medical profession, business executives across the country are—as a group, and especially as purchasers of health care for their employees—withdrawing from the special relationship. Moreover, business executives who maintain the special relationship are unlikely to continue indefinitely separating their sentiments from their practical knowledge, especially as they learn more about the costs of redundant acute care services, overutilization, and the questionable effectiveness of many interventions in both acute and chronic conditions.

By their political behavior, leaders of medicine acknowledge the end of this special relationship. In May 1991, to take a notable instance, executives and officers of the AMA held a press conference in Washington to demand changes in national policy for health care financing. The political news was not that physicians wanted somebody to pay them for treating people who did not have insurance but, rather, that the AMA acted independently of major business associations and of a national administration that was sympathetic to business.[9]

The special relationship began to deteriorate when the business community became concerned about the economy. The recession of 1974 provoked what has turned out to be continuing pessimism in business, government, and the media about declining economic growth, productivity, and competitiveness in world markets. This pessimism intensified and spread throughout the country in the next several years as prices continued to rise faster than real wages and both business and government abolished jobs that had seemed secure.

The cost of health care to employers increased while their receipts and profits diminished, despite the exclusion of employee benefits from taxable corporate income. The more generous the coverage that employers offered, moreover, the greater the incentives that employees had to use health services; and the increased use raised the cost of premiums. Organized labor, especially in the largest industries, had negotiated "first dollar coverage," the removal of any copayments. The absence of copayments accelerated the use of services, rising premiums, and costs to employers.

Employers now paid more attention to the cost of health benefits than they had in more prosperous times. Before the 1970s, business executives usually agreed with physicians that what was technically labeled "medical necessity" drove costs up. Sick people, following the orders and prescriptions of physicians, took appropriate advantage of the latest advances in medical science and technology. Health care was special, as liberals and many economists had argued. Employers now learned, often to their surprise, that health care was a commodity. They acquired some of this learning by reading about physicians' profit seeking in such respected media as the *Wall Street Journal*. Some of it came from observation of or local gossip about lucrative deals between physicians and hospitals.[10] Much of it came about as these employers conducted their businesses, often as they responded to federal policies regulating employee benefits. One such policy was a section of the Employee Retirement and Income Security Act of 1974 (ERISA), which prohibited states from regulating any employment-based benefits except insurance. ERISA preemption, as the policy was called, gave incentives to many large firms to self-insure their employees for health services. Self-insurance almost always saved money for employers, among other reasons because it gave them a direct interest in negotiating discounts from physicians and hospitals.[11] Another instructive federal policy was a section of the Internal Revenue Code, added in 1978, that permitted employees to exercise considerable choice in allocating the income their employers paid them in benefits. As a result of these Cafeteria Plans (and their instruments, Flexible Benefits Accounts), many employees—especially those who were healthier and those who had spouses with family coverage—chose cheaper health coverage and more cash income, often at an overall saving to employers. Employees were regarding health care as just another consumer good.[12]

Employers drew political lessons from their new experience. Self-insurance, like managed care in general, demonstrated that decisions labeled "medically necessary" in fact responded to ordinary economic incentives. Cafeteria Plans made plain that many of the most highly skilled and sought-after workers in the country would exchange increasingly expensive, open-ended medical benefits for cash or for more predictable benefits in kind, such as child care.

In the 1980s, the conservative economists who insisted that health care was a commodity were vindicated by the competitive behavior of many health maintenance organizations, hospital chains, and firms that managed care. Many physicians worked for or owned shares in these organizations, giving business executives additional evidence that physicians responded to economic incentives no differently than they did.

The increasing burden of state and local taxes on business gave executives another reason to reassess their special relationship with physicians. Spending for Medicaid grew faster than any other item in state budgets. Moreover, state and local taxes paid for care in public hospitals and clinics that served people who were not covered by either health insurance or Medicaid. Rising taxes increased the cost of doing business. But interest groups representing health care providers frequently acted in ways that drove taxes up. For example, proposals by governors and legislators to restrict Medicaid coverage or eligibility invariably led to protests from physicians and other health professionals whose

services would be excluded or reduced. In good economic times
and bad, physicians in private practice complained bitterly about
their low reimbursement under Medicaid.

Moreover, increasing numbers of physicians were behaving in
ways that could involve them in conflicts of interest. Such conflicts were hardly new in medicine. At the turn of the century,
when the special relationship between physicians and business
executives began, state medical societies made concerted efforts
to eliminate fee splitting between surgeons and general practitioners and the practice of pharmacy by physicians. Over the next
several decades, the American Medical Association declared that
profit making was "beneath the dignity of professional practice"
but refused to condemn physicians who were owners of proprietary hospitals. Throughout the century, organizations of physicians have insisted that they could manage potential conflicts of
interest by the force of peer pressure and by their domination of
state licensing boards. Medical greed, leaders of the profession
insisted, was deviant behavior, an impairment analogous to, and
sometimes a result of, illness or substance abuse.[13] In the 1970s
and 1980s, however, elite physicians acquired unprecedented incentives to resolve conflicts of interest in their favor. Kenneth
Ludmerer, a physician and historian, writes that medical schools
between the world wars had been a "public trust"; their faculties
"disdained commercialism." The schools would not, for example,
"patent discoveries made by their faculty." In the 1970s, as Ludmerer documents, "changing attitudes towards patients and new
ventures between medical schools and industry sullied the idea
that medical schools are public trusts."[14]

The behavior of academic physicians helped to sanction similar
actions throughout the profession. Summarizing an extensive
study of hospital-physician relationships in ten cities across the
country, sociologist and business school professor Stephen Shortell wrote in 1990 that "hospitals and physicians are beginning to
engage each other as business partners. They are learning more
about each other's legitimate economic interests."[15] Other scholars and journalists documented this partnership. In 1991, a reporter for the *Wall Street Journal* concluded that "free office

space, income guarantees and joint business ventures went a long way toward making doctors think of their interests as being one and the same as the hospitals'.''[16] In 1992, the authors of an article in the *Journal of the American Medical Association* reported that, in Florida, 40 percent of the physicians in direct patient care had an "investment interest in a health care business to which they may refer their patients for services."[17]

Self-policing by the medical profession seemed to be ineffective. Evidence had accumulated since the 1970s that physicians' hearty response to economic incentives was destroying the social contract that medicine and the modern state had negotiated over several centuries. Under this informal contract, physicians had agreed to act at all times in the best interests of their patients. In return, the state gave the medical profession considerable autonomy to decide who could practice and under what standards. Patients ratified this social contract by routinely acting on the advice they received from physicians. Now the autonomy of the medical profession was at risk, and more so in the United States than in any other Western country.[18]

Beginning in the 1970s, powerful people, initially within medicine, claimed that many physicians were violating their fiduciary obligations to their patients. To take perhaps the most prominent example, Arnold Relman, editor of the *New England Journal of Medicine*, complained eloquently, and to great publicity, about a "medical-industrial complex." Relman worried that physicians were purchasing business ventures in diagnostics and surgery and were referring patients to these businesses. Because such referrals increased the cost of care, physicians would further antagonize business and government. Relman and his many supporters advocated remedies that included new law and regulation as well as policing by outside agencies and by physicians themselves.[19]

Officials representing large payers sometimes described the need for a new social contract between physicians and society less diplomatically than Relman and his allies did. For instance, Richard Kusserow, the aggressive inspector general of the Department of Health and Human Services, said, "I do not believe that physicians are less human than other homo sapiens bipeds."[20]

In an attempt to revive the special relationship, leading business executives and prominent health providers established formal "coalitions" in a number of large cities and Washington. Since the 1890s, business executives and physicians had taken their alliance for granted. These coalitions were trying, often lamely, to restore it. In the new coalitions, for example, managers of large hospitals and health care systems often served as surrogates for physicians. The few cities in which an old-style special relationship between business and medicine persisted—for instance, Rochester, New York—received astonished, admiring (and insiders said exaggerated) coverage in the national press.

Neither self-policing nor lawsuits nor attempts at regulation and reconciliation reversed the proliferation of the economic incentives that encouraged significant numbers of physicians to pursue interests that could conflict with the interests and abuse the trust of their patients. For example, Marc Rodwin, a political scientist, presents evidence from court records and other primary sources that physicians have been taking increasing advantage of their opportunities to earn more money.[21]

The malpractice insurance crisis that began in the 1970s contributed to the growing apprehension about physicians' dedication to their patients' interests. Physicians' insurance premiums rose as a result of increasing claims against them and of the rising number and value of settlements and court awards in favor of plaintiffs. Many angry and frustrated physicians blamed the crisis on former allies who had once taken the special relationship for granted. They especially blamed lawyers who took negligence cases for contingent fees and legislators who refused to cap awards by juries for pain and suffering. Many physicians also directed their rage at lawyers and legislators in general. In a 1986 commencement address reported in the *New York Times*, for instance, the president of the Association of American Medical Colleges abused lawyers as sharks.[22] At about the same time, a professional lobbyist hired by the Medical Society of New York State complained to its executive committee that physicians representing the society were insulting legislators at meetings where they were advocating legislation to regulate malpractice litigation.[23]

By the 1990s, physicians were more isolated as a political interest group than they had been at any time since the repeal of state licensing laws during the years of Jacksonian democracy a century and a half earlier. They now had as much political influence as their money could buy, supplemented by the general public's still substantial faith in medical science and its applications.

Disease, Disability, and the Limits of Medicine

Neither economic conditions nor changes in interest group politics alone account for the increasing disarray in health affairs. Since the 1970s, many articulate and influential people have doubted that advances in the science and technology of medical diagnosis and treatment would, by themselves, substantially reduce the burden of chronic disabling illness. Two related ideas encouraged this skepticism about the optimistic promises that physicians and scientists had made to the public and to themselves since the beginning of the century. The first idea was that people's behavior at least partially determines when or whether they will get heart disease, stroke, and certain cancers. The second idea was that, instead of being dichotomously healthy or sick, each person is constantly at risk of disabling illness, or of a worsening of function as a result of a current illness.

Considerable evidence implicated individual behavior in the onset and worsening of many chronic disabling diseases. Beginning with the linkage of smoking and lung cancer in the 1950s, medical scientists demonstrated that what had previously been scientific conjecture or moralizing or folk wisdom (often contradicted by competing wisdom) about how to behave often met the most rigorous tests of contemporary epidemiology. Two decades later, it was hard to avoid knowing that people's decisions about diet, exercise, and the use of tobacco and alcohol influenced what chronic diseases they would get, and when they were likely to get them.

Many medical scientists had been reluctant to explore the association of behavior and illness. They clung to the belief that progress in the struggle against disease would come from laboratory studies of microbes or the degeneration of organ systems. In 1948, for instance, just a few years before epidemiologists established a convincing causal link between cigarette smoking and cancer, John D. Rockefeller, Jr., asked the senior medical executive of the Rockefeller Foundation to explore the feasibility of establishing a substantial research program on the subject. The scientists whom Alan Gregg consulted agreed that "on any scale of values . . . research on the effects of tobacco would come far behind a hundred other studies which would interest good investigators, consume less money and be more likely to be heeded and applied."[24]

Nevertheless, evidence linking behavior and illness accumulated rapidly over the next quarter century, and the American public acted on it. A review in 1989 by James Fries, an influential medical scientist, concluded that since 1953 per capita tobacco consumption had decreased by 40 percent, the use of butter by 33 percent, whole milk and cream by 25 percent, and animal fats and oils by 40 percent. During the same years, consumption of vegetable fats and oils and fish increased by more than 25 percent. Seventy percent of Americans reported that they fastened seat belts in automobiles. These changes in behavior had compellingly strong statistical associations with lower morbidity and, as a result, with a potential reduction in the use of health services and with longer life.[25]

Since the 1950s, clinical epidemiologists have evaluated more systematically than ever before the effectiveness of the treatments prescribed by physicians and other health professionals. A 1984 report by the Office of Technology Assessment of the United States Congress concluded that only about a quarter of standard medical treatments had been subjected to the rigorous methods of randomized controlled trials.[26] In 1989, Congress authorized the Public Health Service to conduct a major research program on medical effectiveness through the new Agency for Health Care Policy and Research. In 1991 and 1992, the Food and Drug Administration announced aggressive new policies for evaluating drugs and devices.

A second challenge to the traditional distinction between health and illness came from new information about the gradual onset of chronic disease and the inability of most treatment to eliminate its underlying pathology. The simplicity and practical importance of distinguishing precisely who was healthy and who was sick had been taken for granted in every area of health policy throughout the century. Researchers studied particular diseases; public health surveillance was based on diagnostic labels; health insurance reimbursed hospitals and physicians for treatments that were based on a precise, numerically coded diagnosis. Patients and most physicians, however, did not sharply differentiate health and illness. Since the 1920s, extensive surveys of the prevalence of morbidity in communities had documented the constant presence of disabling impairments in the lives of a growing number of people.[27] General practitioners' diaries and memoirs reveal that most of their patients complained of recurring and only vaguely diagnosable problems in their joints, lungs, throats, and digestive tracts.

A sharp distinction between health and illness had considerable utility in policy, however. Such a distinction defined the boundaries between health affairs and social policy for welfare and social services, housing, income, and disability. The distinction permitted public agencies and private organizations to measure their work load and justify the resources they wanted or received. The World Health Organization recognized the utility of the distinction in its famous and perhaps idealistic 1946 definition of health as a "state of well-being."[28] Talcott Parsons's classic sociological analysis of the sick role was a commentary on the high value that society assigned to making sharp distinctions between health and illness.

The new evidence that individual behavior determines the onset and course of particular chronic diseases made the conventional distinction between health and illness less useful. Experts, the media, and many individuals themselves now perceived that each person is always at risk, either of acquiring new diseases or of becoming more disabled by existing or latent diseases. Risk is the probability of an event under particular conditions. To be at risk is not to be sick in the conventional sense, since a state of risk is a state in which pathology is absent.[29]

But a century of experience with policy that dichotomized people as either sick or healthy blurred the distinction between being at risk and having a disease. According to political scientist Deborah Stone, who has done pioneering research on this subject, many journalists, policy makers, and members of the public have taken to describing the probabilities of being at risk as if they are "mechanistic causation." Risk factors, she continues, are often misdescribed as "individual traits." Being at risk has become a "form of dangerousness not just to self but to others." Because everyone at risk is a "potential drain on public resources," the new status was becoming a form of "undeservingness" that could justify excluding people from the work force and from entitlement programs.

The at-risk concept could, in the scenarios of some critics, suggest that people with chronic disease are responsible for the failure of a century of promises about the triumphal progress of medical science—promises that had justified health policy for most of the past century. The unwillingness of Americans to use their mouths and muscles the way the new scientific moralizers told them to had outpaced the ability of medical science to cure disease. Americans' reward for believing those promises would, it seemed, be their own disabling chronic diseases. The fault lay not in the promises but in the gullibility and the gluttony—politely labeled inadequate understanding—of those who were propagandized.

Such irony aside, the at-risk concept has profound significance for health policy in the future. If everyone is at some risk of the disabling consequences of chronic illness, the conventional priorities of health policy are obsolete. Decision makers in the public and private sectors now have a long-term financial interest in taking action to reduce risks for individuals and to encourage them to change their behavior. Such actions could prevent or postpone the costs of treating disabling disease. Decision makers also have stronger incentives to make policies that enable people to function more effectively with the disabilities they have, in order to avoid or postpone the progression of disease to stages that are more expensive to manage.[30] The at-risk concept could, therefore, have an additional, even a benign, effect; it could have a better result than the stigmatization and villainization of individuals. The idea that risk is predictable could be the basis of investment in preventive strategies in a troubled economy in which business and public officials are skeptical about the effectiveness and motives of physicians and other health providers.

This conclusion could be too optimistic. The at-risk concept could be stigmatizing if leaders in government and business see no possibility of reducing the enormous costs of acute health services or even their rate of increase. In either event, it will surely matter a great deal in the future that health and illness have become elusive, or even illusory, concepts.

AIDS and the Priorities of Health Policy

The epidemic of AIDS, which was first recognized in 1981, exemplified the disarray in health affairs. Activists accused government agencies, the insurance industry, and many health care providers of withholding resources because most persons with AIDS were homosexuals or intravenous drug users. The evidence suggests a different conclusion. The institutions that implement our health policy responded with alacrity, in accordance with the priorities established and the tools devised during the twentieth century. The response was inadequate not because of who was at risk for the disease but because of the limits of the American health policy compromise.[31]

Most experts first described AIDS to each other and to the media as a plague of acute infectious disease. Decision makers in health affairs had learned to respond to plagues by mobilizing research, treatment, and community resources. Since the nineteenth century, many plagues had come suddenly and then receded, often to return years later. These plagues included cholera, diphtheria, influenza, and polio.

The first evidence that AIDS was a chronic infectious disease, like tuberculosis, rather than a conventional plague, came in 1985 and 1986 as a result of research on cost. Expenditures for treating each person with AIDS were about the same as those for treating persons who had the most prevalent chronic diseases, especially cancer. In what was then an average of eighteen months from diagnosis to death, persons with AIDS used about the same volume of medical, hospital, nursing home, and home-based services that persons with chronic diseases did over a period of approximately a decade. But people in their seventies and eighties incurred most of the costs of treating chronic diseases. Persons with AIDS were typically in their twenties, thirties, or forties.[32]

The negotiators of the health policy compromise had assumed that the most expensive stages of most people's chronic diseases occurred when they were in retirement, either as a result of advanced age or of disability. In retirement, people were eligible for Medicare, the only social insurance program for health care, in which the costs were covered by federal taxes deducted from the paychecks of everyone who worked.

AIDS dramatized problems of voluntary insurance that were already well known to experts and to people who had (or whose dependents had) chronic disabling illnesses that attracted less attention. For example: a few expensive cases of illness in small, experience-rated risk pools made premiums unaffordable; some policies excluded particular chronic diseases; other policies limited coverage, so that benefits were quickly exhausted; most policies did not cover long-term care at all, or covered such care only immediately after hospital stays; people who had recently changed jobs were frequently not covered for preexisting conditions. Medicaid and state or local government became the payers of last resort for persons with AIDS. They already were for everybody else.

Advancing therapeutics provided additional justification for making policy for AIDS as a chronic disease. In 1989, the federal government recommended that persons with HIV take the drug AZT to delay the onset of other infections. Early detection of infection with HIV, monitoring for numbers of T cells, and treatment with AZT and, eventually, other drugs might lengthen the time between infection and death. Within a few months, experts were saying that, with proper treatment, the time from infection to the end stage of the syndrome might soon be eight to ten years.

Defining AIDS as a chronic infectious disease had considerable practical significance. If the Public Health Service had judged the effectiveness of AZT against the criteria for approving antiviral cancer drugs, it would have approved AZT for prophylactic use two years earlier, according to a study by David Rothman and Harold Edgar.[33] Drugs that meet the lower, chronic disease threshold of approval get to patients sooner. Early detection and treatment of AIDS meant, moreover, that considerably more treatment for it would be provided in clinics, physicians' offices, long-term care facilities, and households than in hospitals, where most of the existing treatment programs were based. Redefinition also meant that preventing HIV infection had become a permanent obligation for individuals and for public health agencies.

Persons with HIV infection were now described—by physicians, the media, and often themselves—as suffering from a disabling disease rather than a rapidly fatal affliction. If they were monitored and treated regularly, they could continue to work and to have social lives for years. They could, that is, unless—like many people with other disabling conditions—they were discriminated against. By 1990, shared concern about stigmatization brought together in a political coalition persons concerned about AIDS and members of the disability rights movement.

The Convergence of Health and Disability Policy

Few people in health affairs had paid close attention to the growing political success of the disability rights movement. Since the 1970s, decisions and consent decrees in class action lawsuits on behalf of mentally ill and developmentally disabled persons in several states had improved the quality of care they received. Neonatologists had been confronted by right-to-life and disability rights activists, who insisted on prolonging by any available means the lives of babies born with severe impairments. A few pediatricians and public interest lawyers complained that the federal Supplementary Security Income program and therefore Medicaid discriminated against children because their disabilities were determined by rigid diagnostic criteria rather than by tests of function as they were for adults.[34]

Most people in health affairs ignored or disdained disability policy. Physicians who made determinations of disability under SSI, SSDI, or workers' compensation often regarded this work as poorly paid and demeaning. Managers of hospitals and other facilities regarded Section 504 of the Rehabilitation Act of 1973 as merely another affirmative action program, to be embraced, acquiesced in, or evaded according to local political conditions. Section 504 in fact prohibited discrimination in all situations involving federal funds against "otherwise qualified persons" who had disabling conditions.

In 1983 and 1984, the national controversy over the treatment of Baby Jane Doe made disability policy, and Section 504 in particular, pertinent to a fundamental issue in health policy: who determines what treatment is appropriate? Baby Jane was born with three serious impairments. Right-to-life and disability rights advocates, allied with Reagan administration officials led by Surgeon General C. Everett Koop, insisted to the media and the courts that the baby should undergo intercranial surgery to implant a shunt. Her parents and physicians insisted that conservative treatment with drugs was more appropriate. To obtain better information about the baby's condition, the federal government requested access to her medical record under Section 504. The state of New York, in whose university hospital the baby was being treated, claimed that it had exclusive jurisdiction over the record.[35]

The immediate result of the Baby Jane Doe controversy convinced many people in health affairs that disability policies and their advocates could once again be disregarded. The federal district and appeals courts upheld New York State's denial to the federal government of access to the baby's medical record. Her parents and their physicians also won the media battle. But they won that battle mainly for aesthetic reasons: the media presented the issue as a confrontation between, on one side, an attractive young couple, supported by their parish priest and by soft-spoken young physicians, and, on the other, gray and gruff male lawyers for organizations advocating an absolute right to life.

However, the Baby Jane Doe controversy subsequently became a political victory for the disability rights movement. New federal antidiscrimination legislation and, more important, anxiety to avoid attention from regulators, advocates, and journalists made physicians reluctant to use conservative medical treatment instead of heroic surgical measures. Many hospitals established committees to review decisions made by surrogates and physicians about the treatment of persons with severe disabilities. State protective service agencies developed more effective methods for monitoring hospitals' compliance with Section 504.

The disability rights movement needed allies in health affairs in order to achieve its larger legislative goals. What became the Americans with Disabilities Act of 1990 was drafted in 1986, introduced in Congress in 1987, and endorsed by George Bush during the presidential campaign of 1988. The ADA extended all the protections and most of the penalties of civil rights statutes to persons with disabilities. Its coverage included employment, public accommodations, transportation, and communications.[36] As the bill moved through congressional committees, its supporters claimed that forty-three million Americans would be affected by it, the majority of them people with chronic diseases. Early in the process, the coalition pressing for the ADA embraced activists for many of these diseases, including lobbyists for persons with AIDS.

The ADA is major social policy legislation that was supported by most members of the center-right coalition in Congress as well as by liberals. Cynics attribute much of this support to the fact that the costs of complying with the ADA will be paid primarily by the private sector and by state and local government rather than the federal budget. There is evidence, moreover, that the passage of the ADA may have been influenced by members of Congress and their families who have personal experience with chronic illness and disability.[37]

The ADA's effect on health policy remains uncertain. More

people with chronic disabling diseases are likely to join the labor force as a result of the ADA prohibition of preemployment medical screening. Others are likely to rejoin or remain in it, since employers are now required to make reasonable accommodations in workplace conditions. On the other hand, the ADA permits employers and health insurers to continue to exclude preexisting conditions and deny coverage for particular diseases, as long as these restrictions apply to everyone enrolled in a particular benefit plan. The ADA can also be used to restrict innovation in health policy. In the summer of 1992, the Bush administration denied an application from Oregon for a waiver that would have increased the number of people in the state who received Medicaid. The administration claimed that the waiver was illegal because the ADA prohibits rationing care on the basis of distinctions about the future quality of different persons' lives.

The use of the ADA, as in Oregon, to prevent the placing of limits on access to acute health care could be valuable to provider interest groups eager to preserve the policy priorities of the past. When disability rights advocates claim that denying services to anybody compromises the quality of everybody's life, they offer a convenient rationalization to interests that are eager to expand the supply of health care without restraining the demand for it or making its delivery more efficient. The claim of the disability advocates that limits are always illegal and immoral because someone's care will be limited could become, in practical politics, support for the notion that there is no public interest, only individual interests. Provider groups that have enjoyed the perquisites of the health policy compromise would have no difficulty in accommodating to such a claim.

The ADA could also, and more optimistically, be a guide to how changes in the priorities of health policy might occur. The coalition that passed the ADA made three assumptions. The first assumption is that a large and growing number of persons have chronic disabling conditions. The second is that most of these people want to be productive members of society, but many of them need assistance in order to function according to their capabilities. The final and unproven assumption is that the private and public sectors will pay the costs of implementing the ADA because the results will be satisfying and the penalties for failure appropriate. The future of the coalition will be decided by tests of all three assumptions.

As this chapter has shown, the health politics of the 1990s are the result of twenty years of increasing disarray in health affairs. Many Americans complain about the cost of health care and about the limitations on their access to it, but there is no consensus about solutions to these widely recognized problems. Comparatively few people, either business and political leaders or ordinary voters, endorse policies that require more government control and taypayers' money. Just as few, however, still claim that provider interests are congruent with the public interest.

As this book went to press, a new Democratic administration in Washington had begun to carry out President Clinton's campaign promises for reform in health policy. Optimists in the media and among new political appointees were explaining why the president and his allies in Congress could—in one or two years, or at worst a first term—accomplish reforms in access to health services accompanied by rigorous cost control. Cynics, especially lobbyists for provider and insurance groups, were working to justify their prediction that, once again, the policy compromise would be adjusted, though this time more substantially than at any time since the 1960s.

The theme of this book is that problems that have accumulated in the course of a century cannot be solved quickly. In particular, the long-deferred claims on policy of the burden of chronic disabling illness cannot be addressed by expedients that still accord priority to care for people in acute distress, supplemented by modest coverage for clinical preventive services. The effect on health care costs of an entrenched policy directed at expanding the supply of acute services is unlikely to be reversed by ceilings or global budgets alone, or even by a stipulation that consumers must carry more financial risk for their own care.

The theme of this chapter has been, however, that contemporary disarray in health affairs could become the basis for extensive changes in the priorities of health policy. Making changes in priorities is always painful, especially when those priorities have been justified by beliefs many of us once regarded as self-evidently correct and when they are defended by people who have a great deal at stake and are persuasive, well heeled, and skilled at politics. I turn now to an analysis of some politics and policies that could, eventually, give us a health policy that does more than acknowledge in its rhetoric the burden of chronic illness.

5

Prospects for Policy

For three-quarters of a century, the people who made health policy in the United States accorded priority to acute episodes of illness. They accommodated the disabling consequences of illness and injury within this priority. During the next several decades, policy makers in both government and the private sector will have political and economic reasons to change priorities so that more funds can be allocated to preventing, postponing, and treating chronic illness. They will also be pressed to cap or reduce the overall cost of health care. Despite these reasons and pressures, powerful health care providers will resist substantial changes either in the priorities of health policy or, more important, in the allocation of money to implement them.

What policies are appropriate to the burden of illness on the population? Who can do what to, for, and with whom in order to mobilize support for these policies? I offer some suggestions in this chapter. But first I explore an issue often ignored by people who make recommendations to decision makers: how to increase the likelihood that proposals for reform make political sense and can, therefore, be supported and then implemented by practical men and women who hold public office or lead large corporations, trade associations, unions, and nonprofit organizations.

Ideas and Interests in Making
Practicable Policy

It is not enough to propose a policy because it might solve a
significant problem. In order to be worth making, a proposal
should also be achievable in contemporary American politics.
Many people have made proposals for solving pressing problems
in health affairs. Many people, though fewer, know from experience how health policy is made in the United States. The extraordinarily difficult task is doing both: devising practicable solutions
to solvable problems.

New health policy is made in the United States in response to
power. This power, as I have described in the preceding chapters,
has had two sources, ideas and interests. Adjustments in policy
can be driven by either ideas or interests. Significant changes in
policy occur, as they did early in the century, when ideas and
interests are joined together to address a particular definition of
the problem of illness. Ideas and interests are, in practical affairs,
difficult to separate. I do so here, with deliberate oversimplifica-
tion, to characterize policies that can be enacted and implemented. My examples of the play of ideas and interests in policy
making are taken partly from the literature of political science and
history, but mainly from my firsthand experience in health politics.

A proposed policy has a chance of being enacted if it is attractive to decision makers as an idea. This generalization contradicts
cynical conventional wisdom, which holds that decision makers
act more often on the basis of interests or inertia than on the
merits of ideas. It is, however, supported by research as well as by
the experience of many people I know.[1] Decision makers,
whether in public, commercial, or nonprofit organizations, frequently judge the value of a policy as an idea. They will consider
a proposed policy if it conforms with ideas they have acted on in
the past and if it is supported by colleagues with whom they have
previously agreed. If a proposed policy could be a good idea in
these terms, decision makers will assess the cost, in cash and
conflict, of enacting and implementing it and the benefits it might

confer on people to whom they are accountable. If a proposed policy does not seem, on quick inspection, to be a good idea, decision makers will usually not consider it any further, even if researchers and other experts believe they can prove its value.

In the first two chapters of this book, I described the impact of a self-evident good idea on health policy. About a century ago, many decision makers in the public and private sectors accepted the idea that increasing the supply of hospitals, physicians, and medical research would eventually make people healthier, because it would alleviate the acute symptoms of illnesses that were mainly the result of infections. For most of the next century, these decision makers and their successors implemented this idea in their policies, at considerable cost to philanthropists and taxpayers.

Then I described evidence that this idea did not adequately take into account the growing incidence and prevalence of chronic disabling illness. For a variety of reasons, decision makers made reducing the burden of chronic illness a high priority in research policy, but they did not give comparable priority to supplying facilities and professionals or to financing health services directed at treating chronic illness.

Decision makers often rely on ideas about governance and process as criteria for accepting or rejecting a proposal for new policy. For instance, many decision makers believe that most direct-service programs run by a government agency will be poor programs even when they are continuously scrutinized. Both the health policy compromise that I described in chapter 3 and the conservative resurgence that I presented in chapter 4 relied heavily on this idea. Decision makers will create and maintain these direct-service programs only when they see no effective alternatives and when they have been persuaded that the benefits the programs confer outweigh the costs of vigilance. Hospitals and nursing homes for veterans of foreign wars are examples of public direct-service programs that have remained attractive by this criterion. In contrast, public acute care hospitals have become unattractive in many cities and states during the past generation. All over the country, public hospitals have been closed or transformed into nonprofit or even investor-owned institutions.[2]

The actual benefits of a policy that decision makers consider an attractive idea can be deferred almost indefinitely. This point again contradicts cynical wisdom, which is that people who make decisions, especially if they hold elective office, want immediate results—if not now, at least in time for the next election. But until very recently, immediate results were not expected from a policy to subsidize research in biomedical science; that research was not expected to produce measurable benefits in health status or economic growth in a particular period of time. In contrast, advocates of a policy to provide more prenatal care for pregnant women eligible for Medicaid (a less attractive idea that was, of course, supported by weaker organized interests) were unsuccessful until they promised to obtain specific results in a specific time period. During the 1980s, they promised that this policy would lead to better birth outcomes, measured by more children being born at term and at higher weight, and to actual cost savings within a few years; moreover, the data they furnished to support their promise were endorsed and augmented by the National Academy of Sciences and leading pediatricians. Only then was the policy enacted.

As I mentioned earlier and as this example demonstrates, ideas and interests can never be entirely separate in political affairs. I separate them temporarily here in order to analyze the political feasibility of proposed policies. For example, because many people who live in rural areas accept ideas that have been in good standing throughout this century, they assume that closing the small general hospitals that serve their communities would endanger their health. They agree so strongly with this idea that most of the men and women they elect to public office regard it as stupid politics to present them with the considerable data to the contrary.[3] Compare this situation with that of people in another rural community that is adjacent to an obsolete and almost empty state mental hospital. Since their stake in the hospital is entirely economic and not rooted in ideas about their health, elected officials can sometimes be persuaded to discuss converting it into a prison or a geriatric center or a community college.

Ideas about acute care have an enormous effect on what policy can be made about managing chronic illness and disability. Decision makers, and not just rural legislators, frequently assert that any reduction in spending to treat acute illness would have adverse effects on health status and that these effects would quickly become apparent to many people. They therefore assume that funds for managing chronic illness must be added to, rather than reallocated within, the overall health care budget. This assumption translates into policy that directly and indirectly imposes a budgetary ceiling on services for chronic illness and disability in both the public and private sectors.

The idea that funds cannot be redirected from acute to chronic care without causing harm is contradicted by substantial evidence. According to some researchers, such redistribution could produce benefits without having adverse effects. Studies of treatment for several chronic diseases that absorb billions of dollars— diabetes and asthma, for instance—conclude that changes in how physicians treat patients could result in considerable savings in acute care, and particularly in hospital, costs.[4] A study of care for a variety of chronic conditions convinced some experts, according to an editorial in the *Journal of the American Medical Association*, that "broadly trained generalists appear to be more parsimonious in their use of medical resources" for patients with chronic diseases than "their more narrowly trained specialty colleagues."[5] Some studies are even more specific, describing diagnostic procedures that lead to acute interventions that are "unnecessary, or at least could be postponed."[6] An increasing number of controlled studies with large samples conclude that some acute interventions are harmful as well as expensive.[7]

But such evidence on behalf of redistributing resources within health care has not been translated into what most leaders in government and business regard as good ideas. Why it has not is open to debate. A contributory cause is certainly the adamant opposition to redistribution among most lobbyists for hospitals and organizations of physicians. I will return later in this chapter to the practical problem of mobilizing support for policies that are repugnant to powerful interest groups.

Because of the strong credibility of the idea that the costs of acute care cannot be reduced without causing harm, we have had a highly emotional, skewed, and perhaps unnecessary national debate about rationing. There has been a great deal of public discourse about whether and how to ration intensive care and other acute interventions, especially for persons who are terminally ill (the euphemism is ''have a poor prognosis'') or who may be labeled by others as expecting a diminished quality of life.

The most frequently debated questions, whether and how to ration care for persons who are terminally ill, are riveting, but they may be tangential to the politics of changing priorities. Just as there is growing evidence that redistributing funds from acute to chronic services or from specialists to generalists causes more good than harm, there are suggestive data that the debate about the costs of terminal care is more symbolic than real. There is, for example, much anecdotal evidence that physicians, often with consent from patients and their families, already reduce the intensity of care for patients who have poor prognoses. In a quantitative study conducted at the Palo Alto Clinic, Ann Scitovsky found that care ''embodied rational constraints for patients with poor prognoses.'' A national study of longitudinal data completed in 1992 offered guarded support for these findings, but concluded that the ''absolute level of services used by persons with chronic impairment over an extended period of time is probably high relative to the likely benefit from the services.''[8]

Translated into practical politics, this evidence may mean that we do not have to engage in endless, and probably fruitless, debate about whether and how to ration care at the end of life. Americans may be limiting their consumption of useless and expensive services at the end of their lives by asserting their values. That is how patients, families, and professionals already behave in most other industrial countries.

If we can cease the aggravating and sterile debate about rationing at the end of life, we may be able to make policy to replace the rationing by default that our institutions have condoned for three-quarters of a century. What we frequently and effectively ration for most persons with chronic illnesses is not acute care but, rather, services that could enhance their independence and productivity. The services we ration include professional assistance in rehabilitation, clinical preventive services, long-term care, and personal assistance with the activities of daily living. We ration these services by leaving much of the need for them uncovered by public or private insurance and by not giving them priority in subsidies for facilities, professional education, and research.

Such rationing has been an unplanned rather than a deliberate result of policy. Because decision makers assume that reducing expenditures for acute care will cause catastrophes, they take actions that, in effect, withhold care from persons with chronic illness until its absence makes them eligible for acute services, for institutionalization, or for both. The compelling, but perhaps obsolete, idea that we should not (or that we cannot) reduce resources for acute care is the most important legacy of the consensual health policy created at the last turn of the century. The idea that acute care costs cannot be reduced is reinforced by the practice of defensive medicine; physicians fear that their risk of being sued increases when they practice conservatively. Moreover, in the absence of rationing or better counseling, patients often self-refer themselves for expensive acute services.

A related idea, beloved by some economists and many provider groups, is the woodwork metaphor. This is a futilitarian justification for covert rationing of care for chronic illness. Its advocates claim that any preventive service or any intervention that permits people to function more effectively will be more expensive to society because more people will demand it. Proponents of the woodwork metaphor assume, however, that the supply of acute services (relative to the size and age of the population) can never decline and that there are no measurable limits to the health services people will demand when the services are accessible. Both of these assumptions could be shaky. Moreover, some practical people in government and business might be persuaded to try making policy on a fresh idea that contradicts the woodwork metaphor. This new idea is that any expensive acute service that can be postponed for a year or longer because of a preventive or supportive service provided today might be paid in a different fiscal climate, or at least by different people.

Sometimes ideas that are significant in general political discourse influence health policy only because advocates mobilized support for them. In the 1890s, for instance, advocates for new priorities in health policy linked them to the prevailing idea in religious doctrine that rich people had a moral obligation to give to charity, that they were stewards of wealth. Within a few years, wealthy donors, as individuals and through philanthropic foundations, provided unprecedented amounts of money for building and staffing hospitals and medical research laboratories.

Two ideas that have recently been transferred to health policy from other arenas have powerful advocates: the notion that health care is a commodity and the concept of autonomy. In the 1960s and 1970s, some economists and their supporters among libertarians introduced the idea that the health sector is a market and that its services are commodities. During the same years, not entirely by coincidence, medical ethicists—a label used by assorted clergy, philosophers, physicians, and advocates for women and minorities—persuaded many people to value the concept of autonomy, or the primacy of the individual, more highly than that of beneficence in the relationship between health professionals and patients. Ethicists and economists who rejected the idea that individuals or social groups can act effectively in the interests of others sometimes disparaged the concept of beneficence, doing good for others, as paternalism. As a result of the idea that health care is a commodity, discourse about policy now routinely uses the words *consumers* and *providers, costs* and *benefits.* The idea of autonomy gave new meaning to the informed consent requested by physicians from patients before performing invasive procedures or using them as subjects in research. Blended, the two ideas stimulated new attention to consumer choice and patients' rights, issues that matter a great deal to policy directed at chronic illness.

Thus, ideas matter to policy makers, but these ideas matter most when they satisfy interests, a subject that I now address in more detail. Most people believe that they know about interests and interest groups without having to read research reports on these subjects. They know about interests when their jobs or the value of their homes is threatened or when a child or aged parents need long-term care. Moreover, most people spend money, time, or just their votes anticipating threats to their interests. More than thirty million people over the age of fifty, to take just one example, believe that membership in the American Association of Retired Persons is cheap at the price.

Nevertheless, people who work for powerful interest groups and those who study them have additional knowledge. Most important, they know that political alliances are fragile and that no group ever owns an important public official, or not for very long. Although the fragility of alliances is a constant of politics, it is usually impossible to predict what changes will occur. Since the 1920s, for instance, scholars and journalists have described the attitudes and behavior of members of the interest groups in health affairs. None of them, however, anticipated the breakdown of the special relationship between physicians and business executives that has occurred in the past decade and a half.

Alliances can be made and maintained for particular purposes by groups that oppose each other on many other matters. In 1974, for instance, a conference committee of the House and Senate, resolving disputed issues in a bill about pensions, prohibited the states from regulating any employer-provided fringe benefits that were not insurance. This prohibition (called preemption) was promoted by both organized labor and the major business associations. They have protected it ever since, despite attempts by other powerful groups, endorsed by influential members of Congress and recently by the National Governors' Association, to change it.[9]

Experts on interest groups, in politics, journalism, or social science, frequently underestimate the power of new alliances. A recent book documents the surprise of John F. Kennedy's advisers in 1961 when they discovered that public opinion strongly supported creating health insurance for the elderly under Social Security.[10] A political scientist, in a major treatise on disability policy, predicted that the Americans with Disabilities Act could not be enacted; six months later, it was.[11]

Decision makers who have a power base and therefore continuing importance are rarely captives of any interest group. Very few legislators believe that their seat is safe, whatever their seniority and margin of victory in the last election. Legislators always run scared. Because they do, they test every proposed policy, not only for its merits as an idea but also for its conformity with the interests of their constituents. Smart interest group leaders try to influence legislators who have many constituents who share the position they advocate. Few campaign contributions could be large enough to persuade a rural Republican to vote consistently for expanding Medicaid eligibility or services for the urban poor. On the other hand, conservative legislators from the suburbs have responded favorably when busloads of their constituents employed by a Medicaid clinic protested against its closure.

Decision makers in the executive branch of federal and state government also know how to distance themselves from interest group pressures. These officials, senior staff to governors and presidents, know from experience that interest groups always want more money and protection, that the agency heads who report to them unofficially encourage private groups to lobby on their behalf, and that every executive agency has an internal imperative toward growth in good economic times and immunity to retrenchment in bad. They have many techniques for evading these pressures.

However, neither legislators nor executive branch officials like to support a new policy if it has conspicuous enemies who make contributions to political campaigns or who have access to the media. Legislators are even more wary of controversy than senior executives are. Conflicts over policy in legislatures are usually won, in the end, by enormous majorities, however closely divided legislators have been in committee. Close votes make incumbents more vulnerable targets for angry interest groups. For instance, Medicare was passed by a large majority in 1965, but only after important groups of physicians signaled that their opposition was no longer based on fundamental principles. The administration had supported it long before. A huge number of voters and a majority of the members of Congress also had supported it for several years. In our time, abortion rights and reform in health care financing have been held hostage by powerful interest groups.

I know less from firsthand experience about the political behavior of business executives than I do about those in government and interest groups. My observation and conversations suggest that there are many similarities among them. New ideas make sense to people in business, as they do to people in government, when their peers find them acceptable. It seems to be as uncomfortable for persons in business as it is for those in government to be perceived as outliers. Thus, in all sectors, it seems safer to support existing policies until a large number of people support proposed changes in these policies.

For a long time, leaders in business, like those in government, left the controversial subject of health policy to the experts. Like their counterparts in government, however, business leaders are wary of experts; and most of them acknowledge and therefore can resist the temptation to become partially informed pseudo-experts themselves.

The purpose of the preceding discussion was to create a context for assessing practical policies in the remaining pages of this book. I sought to reassure experts on politics that I know firsthand how difficult it is to make and implement policy and to introduce other readers to some of the problems of making public decisions.

Policy innovation in health affairs is possible, but only if a number of conditions are met. The most important of these conditions are the following:

- The idea embodied in the policy appears capable of producing measurable benefits for identifiable people in a period of time that politically significant numbers of people consider reasonable.
- The idea resonates with other ideas that have generally favorable connotations among decision makers.
- Interest groups that have significant resources and influence support the idea, while other powerful groups are afraid to oppose it vigorously.
- Powerful people in the legislative and executive branches of government and in the private sector see

sufficient merit in the idea, and enough public support
for it, to ignore or challenge colleagues and powerful
interests that actively oppose it.

Current Proposals to Reform
Health Care Financing

Most of the proposals for reform in national health policy that are
now under consideration by the media, interest groups, the administration, and Congress do not change the priority accorded to
chronic disease and disability. Each of the leading proposals
would increase the number of people who have access to acute
inpatient and hospital services and to some preventive services.
Each has mechanisms to slow the rate at which costs increase. A
few proposals would cover more services, especially long-term
care, for persons with chronic disease and disability. But these
proposals avoid the issue of priority by simply increasing the overall cost of health care. Priorities are notoriously difficult to change.
Contemporary health policy is the result of almost a century of
accretion. The compromise negotiated in the 1950s and 1960s was
possible only because the priorities of health policy established
during the previous half century became self-evident ideas that
had, over time, acquired support among decision makers and
leaders of interest groups of providers, purchasers, and even consumers of services.

Practical people who want to change the priority accorded to
chronic disabling illness and injury are most likely to succeed
eventually if they first support policies to improve access to acute
services—policies such as increasing the number of people who
have insurance coverage for routine acute and preventive services; increasing the average size of the groups over which risks
and costs are spread or just eliminating small groups; and setting
budget caps and ceilings in order to restrain cost increases. These
policies could be achieved by a variety of means. Any feasible
proposal would, however, probably preserve a strong private sector of payers and providers; limit patients' ability to choose provid-

ers without eliminating it entirely; and create incentives to reduce administrative costs, including the cost of regulation.

Many public officials and leaders of interest groups now agree that the current policy compromise needs to be adjusted. Each time there was such near unanimity in the past, adjustment has occurred. History never repeats itself, or only with variations that make prediction impossible. But assume for a moment that some adjustment in the compromise is likely to occur in the next several years and that, as a result, it will then become feasible to think of ways to accord higher priority to preventing and managing chronic disabling illness and injury. It is also prudent to assume that the politics of improving access to acute care in the mid-1990s will be bitter and therefore exhausting. Consequently, there may be no opportunity for many years to conduct a well-publicized debate about adjusting priorities in order to use more resources to prevent and manage chronic illness and disability.

Debates about adjusting the American health policy compromise have always been replete with exaggerations and distortions of fact and have created bitterness that limits subsequent reform. A famous example of residual bitterness occurred in 1965 and 1966 when many physicians opposed Medicare and Medicaid on ideological grounds. Rage prevented most of them from noticing that their fee schedules and professional dominance had been protected by the new federal legislation. As a result, they did not immediately calculate the extent to which these programs, Medicare especially, would improve their incomes. At the same time, their opposition to Medicare before its passage persuaded most leaders of Congress and the executive branch that it would be bad politics to promote additional increments of reform. Their liberal reformist colleagues who insisted that national health insurance, in some form, was "imminent" were, as events soon made plain, out of touch with health politics.

Information is still distorted by all sides in debates about health policy. If adjustments in the compromise are made in the 1990s, their political cost could once again polarize interest groups and prevent serious negotiations about priorities. In a political atmosphere in which words like *socialized medicine, Canadian health care, rationing,* and even *taxation* and *family* have acquired almost entirely symbolic meanings, it may be difficult to engage decision makers in sustained discussion about people with chronic illness.

New Priorities of Policy

Assume that in the mid-1990s some combination or modification of current proposals for reforming access to health care and for capping or controlling costs becomes national policy or is adopted by many states. The number of people without any health insurance or the equivalent could be sharply reduced. People who want the most comprehensive insurance coverage could pay more for it, in some combination of higher premiums and more of their income that is taxable. People with preexisting chronic diseases could not be denied coverage or be required to wait before insurance would pay for their care. Employees of small firms could no longer be threatened with sudden increases in their health insurance premiums when one or a few fellow workers became seriously and chronically ill. People could change jobs without fear of losing coverage for themselves and their families.[12]

If several of these changes occur in policy for access, they would almost certainly be accompanied by new measures to control cost. These measures would probably restrain demand for health services. Such policies could include, for example, higher deductibles and coinsurance, more effective utilization review, and managed care, in several of its variants.

A reasonable next step would be to reshape health policy so that it takes explicit account of the pressure of chronic disabling illness and injury. I propose two goals for policy. The first goal is a politically painful precondition of the second. It is to redistribute some of what we now spend for infrequently used or redundant acute care services in order to manage more effectively the consequences of chronic disabling illness and injury. As redistribution proceeds, we should, as the second goal, make policy to spend the reclaimed money on efforts to postpone or prevent the onset of disease, reduce or eliminate the risk of injury, and prevent the disabling consequences of illness and injury for individuals from getting worse.

Redistribution is necessary and practical. Much of the money for preventing and managing the consequences of chronic illness and injury can come from within the health sector.[13] Although experts fight about the precise numbers, hardly anybody disagrees that the people of most other industrial democracies are at least as healthy as we are, and that these countries spend a lower percentage of their national income on personal health services than the United States does. Moreover, there are persuasive arguments that spending for health care is not as advantageous to the economy as other expenditures.[14] Americans have a great deal they want to do with their incomes, collectively and individually, besides pay for health services.

If redistribution should occur, the hospital industry would lose most of its current excess capacity; and more of its capacity would become redundant as more chronic illness is prevented or postponed. At any moment in recent years, about 40 percent of the acute general hospital beds in the country have been staffed and empty, at an annual cost that was calculated, controversially, in 1992 to be about twelve billion dollars. About 30 percent of the capacity of the one thousand smallest general hospitals is used for the same purposes that are served—at a lower cost—by nursing homes and sometimes home health care.[15] But many people have big stakes in maintaining the hospital industry at or near its present state of readiness for acute intervention. Redistribution would mean that hospitals and the firms that supply and equip them would lose employees. In some communities, the loss of hospital-related jobs would make a bad situation worse. For example, since 1991, the hospitals of Flint, Michigan, have employed more people than the city's General Motors plants.[16] Many medical schools and teaching hospitals also would be losers; they are major suppliers of acute services and of the highly skilled professionals who do the most expensive diagnoses, intensive care, and surgery. Because of these stakes, it is not surprising that hospital leaders all over the country are claiming that their institutions are or should be major providers of primary care for their communities. Physicians and hospital managers are embracing the rhetoric of new priorities, and of course some of the substance, in order to protect their existing interests.

A second target of redistribution is medical specialty services and, over time, our excessive number of highly specialized physicians. In comparison with Western European countries or Canada, we have too many subspecialists and too few primary care practitioners. Studies that rely entirely on domestic evidence reach the same conclusion. Even free-market advocates agree that the current distribution of physicians among specialties is mainly a result of market failure. We have too many specialists because the states, the federal government, and private insurers subsidize their residency and training and because, traditionally, specialists receive higher fees than primary care physicians.

The United States needs a medical equivalent of arms control in international affairs (or, in a more contentious metaphor, of birth control). The production of physicians who perform the most expensive diagnostic and therapeutic procedures, and who use the most expensive equipment, needs to decrease. Such a decrease would be particularly welcome among specialists who perform procedures that frequently turn out to be unnecessary or potentially harmful. At the same time, the number of physicians who assist their patients in managing chronic disabling illness and injury should increase.

The redistribution I propose could happen only gradually. Over several years, for example, funds could be removed from the support of hospitals and training for some medical specialties and transferred to care in the community that would reduce the burden of chronic illness.

I will discuss the politics of redistribution in the final section of this chapter. My purpose now is to suggest how to use some of the reclaimed funds to meet the related goals of managing and preventing disability that results from chronic illness and injury.

Management and prevention are inseparable. Almost everyone agrees that any disease or injury that can be prevented should be prevented. Only a few modern Malthusians, along with some of the people I have been calling futilitarians, worry that we would then incur more costs for income and services to the elderly, because people would survive to old age in greater numbers. Moreover, with the exception of a few diseases, like chicken pox, which are more dangerous in adults than in children, any affliction that can be postponed until later in life should be postponed.

Diseases and injuries will happen, of course, in spite of our efforts to prevent or postpone their onset. Therefore, the priority of health and related services must be to manage the consequences of disease and injury. Managing illness has conventionally meant alleviating pain and postponing particular impairments and the moment of death. This definition of management has been expanding to include preventing people's existing impairments from disabling them further.

In the discussion that follows, I separate the management of illness from the prevention of illness mainly because many people currently think of them as different aspects of health care. For clarity, I begin by considering management in its narrowest definition: providing diagnostic and treatment services to a particular person.

According higher priority to management would mean that more professionals spend more time talking with patients. Talk that is pertinent to managing chronic illness and injury includes advice about preventing or postponing disease; history-taking that helps the professional make early diagnoses; assistance in behavior modification; education in treatment regimens; and discussion of the consequences of choices that could reduce disability—for example, choices among drugs, devices, and modifications of home and workplace. But more than talk is necessary. Many people require assistance in accommodating to their impairments. Some of this assistance could be provided by professionals, especially by physicians, nurses, physical and occupational therapists, social workers, and job counselors. Much assistance, however, is not currently within the domain of health policy. Such assistance includes personal care, income support, and disability management in the workplace. Personal care means assistance, beyond what members of a household can provide, in carrying out the usual activities of daily life. Income support, in practical terms, means the inclusion of temporary and partial disabilities in Social Security Disability Insurance (disabilities now excluded from SSDI). Disability management in the workplace means accommodating settings, equipment, and work rules to the mutual advantage of employer and employee.

Managing chronic disease and injury requires that more provision be made for long-term care. But how much long-term care, where it would be provided, and how much it would cost can only be conjectured. For example, future policy could promote the establishment of more extended households, in which people help each other manage the consequences of chronic disabling illness and injury, thereby reducing their dependence on professional services. Current examples of such households include independent living centers and various types of congregate living arrangements for elderly people and persons with developmental disabilities and mental illness.

Prevention will have the most important, and unpredictable, influence on demand for long-term care. Acute care that is avoided or postponed does not require convalescence. Disabling conditions that can be accommodated in households and workplaces will not require institutionalization. On the other hand, demand for personal services, both nonmedical and medical, is likely to increase if people lead longer, more productive, and more independent lives. Whether there is money to meet that demand will depend largely on how successfully policy can restrain entrepreneurs who are eager to increase, and profit from, the supply of services.

Prevention, whether it is conceived as part of the management of illness and injury or as a separate set of activities, is currently being redefined. For the past century, the priority of prevention policy has been to reduce the number of new cases of disease—primarily through surveillance of populations and patients, immunization, sanitation, and the treatment and segregation of persons with contagious diseases. Prevention policy, that is, has been the responsibility of public health agencies in the states and local communities. Clinical prevention has most often consisted mainly of immunizing patients against infectious diseases.

Since the 1960s, policy to prevent illness has given increasing emphasis to chronic disease. Considerable funds have been spent to persuade people to change their behavior, especially in regard to smoking, exercise, diet, and the use of alcohol and addictive drugs. Policy to regulate hazardous substances that cause chronic disease, in the workplace and communities, has become more important than it was earlier in the century.

Policy for prevention has also been according higher priority to the disabling consequences of illness and injury. An international nomenclature that has gained many adherents, especially in Europe, since it was devised in the late 1970s makes a useful distinction among impairments, disabilities, and handicaps. According to this scheme, impairments are disturbances in the processes or the structures of the body as a result of inheritance (or birth), disease, or injury. Disabilities are particular limitations in activity as a result of impairment. Handicaps are the social disadvantages that result from impairment and disability.[17]

The new classification, according to its creators and advocates, facilitates changing the priorities of policy because it makes explicit an important conceptual change: it links anatomical or mental pathology as a result of chronic disease to human behavior. For the first time, decision makers and health professionals have a method to describe, and keep accurate records about, what impairments people have and what is done to prevent the worsening of disabilities and handicaps that result from them. In combination with rapidly evolving methods for assessing the results, or outcomes, of intervention, the classification is potentially a powerful tool for decision makers and health professionals.[18]

A change in priorities for prevention policy would have many practical consequences, only a few of which can be anticipated. Traditional public health measures for preventing impairment would still be necessary, especially for preventing impairment that results from infections and from diseases and injuries that can be avoided by personal behavior. But policy would have to give new priority to interventions that are not currently in the mainstream of medical practice. Some of these changes—for example, improving and distributing devices that increase the functional capacity of persons whose mobility or sensory abilities are impaired—would cost money. Wheelchairs and motorized carts, for instance, have had such a low priority in policy that what seems to be the only systematic published comparison among competing models was made by the editor of a popular automotive magazine, who is a wheelchair user.[19]

Others changes in prevention policy could make available for redistribution funds currently spent on pensions and on care that is mainly custodial. A substantial number of people with disabling conditions tell researchers and testify to legislative hearings that they are eager to be employed or to remain in their jobs. The work rules and physical environment of many workplaces can be modified to enable persons with disabling conditions to gain or retain employment. There is evidence that the cost of these accommodations in the workplace offsets some of the cost of public programs for income replacement and medical care.[20]

The changes in policy that I am suggesting will require considerable investment in research. Much more needs to be understood about the causes and processes of impairment and about the effectiveness of competing measures for preventing disability. Some redistribution of resources may result from research that suggests measures of acute intervention that are ineffective. But most medical researchers outside the field of clinical epidemiology are likely to ally with the opponents of changes in priorities, for reasons I now address as part of a broader exploration of the politics of redistributing what we now spend on health care.

The Politics of Establishing New Priorities

New priorities can be set only if new political alliances are formed. Who, at a minimum, would have to agree? Who is friendly to revising the priorities of health policy? Who is an enemy or a potential enemy? How could new allies overcome opposition to changing the priorities of policy?

Americans may become receptive to new priorities for health policy. Opinion surveys have documented increasing concern about health care in representative samples of the public. The media and official public hearings have offered considerable anecdotal evidence about these concerns. In casual conversation, almost every American over the age of forty tells personal anecdotes about getting assistance for a person with a chronic disabling condition. But most Americans are more likely to support than to press actively for change. Health policy is not the highest priority for most people. Few of us will attend a meeting, write a letter, or cast a vote on behalf of policy that could raise our taxes or reduce our take-home pay. Because a large number of Americans work in the health sector, moreover, almost everybody who does not has a relative or a friend who could lose a job if the priorities of policy change.

A coalition that could bring about significant change must have considerable strength among organizations that pay for health care. The coalition would have to include employers with a variety of employees: young as well as middle-aged and both stable and transient. It would also have to include the leading firms in the health insurance industry as well as large Blue Cross plans and health maintenance organizations, organized labor, governors, state legislators, and powerful members of Congress. Even this alliance might not be able to reach agreement on overall policy unless a president of the United States is willing to take political risks to change priorities in health policy.

Most interest groups in health affairs are unlikely to support new priorities unless a coalition led by payers appears to be on the verge of victory. Hospital associations, traditionally dominated by the institutions' chief executive officers, have almost always acted on behalf of their members' economic interests; the newly formed associations of trustees have yet to take independent political action. The proprietors of nursing homes and home health care agencies and the manufacturers of most drugs, supplies, and equipment have a huge economic stake in chronic illness. But they now depend on hospitals for most of their business.

Associations of health care practitioners have many reasons to oppose changing priorities. Most physicians, even those in primary care and specialties that treat chronic diseases, still regard professional solidarity as vital to their self-esteem and political

interests. Medical scientists and specialists who do invasive procedures have for a long time considered themselves superior to
physicians who provide primary care or take care of patients with
lingering chronic diseases. Most of these physicians learned in
medical school and residency training to feel superior to colleagues in public health and preventive medicine. Organizations
of nurses and allied health professions have frequently advocated
that more services be available for persons with chronic illness.
But they will not endorse redistribution that could threaten their
incomes and access to supervisory positions or their fragile status
in universities.

If the politics are managed adroitly, however, some physicians
and other health professionals could join alliances for change, or
at least not actively oppose them. Health professionals are, in
general, eager to satisfy their patients. An ideology of concern for
patients is central to the training and practice of each health
profession. Like any ideology, this one has aspects that are self-
serving and contradictory. But patient-centeredness has recently
been accorded new practical significance as a result of increased
competition among providers and of payment policies that take
account of data about patients' satisfaction with their treatment.

Assume for a moment that in the next several years reforms,
national or state by state, are made in policy for access to basic
health services, and that a coalition for changing priorities can be
established. The members of the coalition should work to redistribute expenditures from the supply of acute care services to the
prevention and management of chronic illness and injury. As decision makers in the countries of the European Community discovered in the 1980s, reducing the supply of acute care services is
usually the most effective method to slow growth in the total cost
of health care.[21]

The principal targets for redistribution, as I described above,
are specialized medical care and hospital services. Feasible goals
would be to change the current ratio of subspecialists to primary
care physicians and to reduce the number of acute hospital beds:
the ratio might drop from three to one to perhaps one to one over
several decades; the number of beds could drop by almost 40

percent in the same period. Potentially effective policies to reduce the ratio of subspecialists to generalists could include the reallocation of subsidies by the states to public medical schools and teaching hospitals; action by the insurance industry, the federal government, and the states to reduce reimbursement to hospitals for the cost of graduate medical education in particular specialties; and new state licensing requirements that restrict entry to particular specialties.[22] Some hospitals and beds could be eliminated as a result of reimbursement policy; others could be eliminated if state and local subsidies for tax-exempt bonds were withheld or if trustees could be persuaded to act on behalf of their communities, rather than as agents for maintaining or increasing the earnings and job satisfaction of physicians, hospital managers, and their suppliers.

The coalition should give priority to policy that changes the boundaries between the acute general hospital and other settings for providing care. The amount of surgery and diagnostic radiology conducted in ambulatory settings has increased in the past decade. Average hospital stays have declined in response to pressure from payers and the introduction of new technology. There is considerable evidence that the number and size of hospitals could be reduced at a faster rate and that physicians could substitute effective lower-cost technologies for many invasive procedures. Moreover, if the affordability and availability of home care and congregate living increased, many patients could be discharged sooner from hospitals. What has been missing is effective political action to change the acute general hospital's role in the provision of health services.[23]

Resistance to carrying out these recommendations will become vicious. Providers will retaliate to threats of cuts or caps by offering gruesome evidence that retrenchment causes people to suffer pain or death. Throughout the country, people will see and hear threats in the media that they will have to wait hours, days, or even months to see a physician, even when they are in pain. Evidence alleged to be relevant will be presented, often out of context, from Western Europe, Canada, and Japan. Defenders of health care policy in other countries will be quoted making statements that sound anti-American. Medical educators and hospital administrators will insist that, with fewer physicians training in the subspecialties of medicine and surgery, they will be unable to give proper care to the poor, especially in cities. Providers and their allies in the interest groups and government will talk about economic dislocation, especially lost jobs, and the betrayal of community traditions.

Such arguments have been made, effectively, many times in the recent past. At a former place of employment, an academic medical center, I helped organize successful defenses against state policies that aimed to slow growth in the number of subspecialists and beds for acute care. I helped to make, and sometimes thought I believed, most of the retaliatory arguments in the preceding paragraph.

There is no unambiguous evidence, however, from anywhere in North America or Europe, that deliberately reducing the supply of acute services, especially hospital facilities and the services of specialized physicians, has had adverse effects on morbidity and mortality in the population. Moreover, most of the horrible instances of neglected or abused or merely waiting patients that are used by provider interest groups defending against cuts actually occur every day, even when cuts are not threatened.

A coalition that presses to redistribute resources in order to prevent, postpone, and manage chronic illness and disability would, moreover, have a political advantage that previous budget cutters lacked. The coalition could promise real benefits to identifiable individuals. Most people have only an abstract interest in cost containment, and none at all when they are sick. However, they could become interested in redistributing resources if they knew that the redistribution would make specific services available to prevent or treat illnesses that they or their relatives have or are likely to have. To show people that they have a personal interest in redistribution, to encourage them to support it actively in order to become "empowered," will require changing some of the conventional rhetoric and practices of health politics. Instead of struggling to answer the dramatic question about life support—"Who shall live?"—leaders of a new coalition need to insist that a more practical question is "How shall we live?" or, more specifically, "How shall we take care of ourselves and each other when, as is inevitable, our impairments make us unable to live as we would choose?"

Most Americans will live longer than most of the people who preceded them. But the overall ratio of births to deaths will remain one to one, as a professor of medicine is alleged to have said earlier in this century, in order to challenge his students' naive enthusiasm about progress. The priority of policy ought to be to postpone disease, prevent injury, and accommodate to disability.

A coalition that wants to change the priorities of health policy would promote the notion that while we appreciate the policies that took us this far, we need new ones. Public education is essential for political success. The policies that need to be modified have been in place for a long time. They provide many people with secure and often very satisfying jobs; some people live very comfortably as a result of these policies. Moreover, a great many members of the public are easily frightened by threats to remove or reduce or make less accessible facilities for acute health services, even when these facilities are redundant by every measure except those used by providers.

Changes of the scope I am recommending would require leaders in economic affairs, government, and, eventually, provider groups to revise fundamental assumptions about health policy. For a century, health policy has been dominated by providers, especially by physicians. Most leaders in business, labor, and government agreed with the priorities and policy choices of health care providers. As a result, health policy was made, most of the time, by relatively small groups of people who were well aware of each other's competing and congruent interests.

Health policy was usually made, moreover, by people who knew little and cared less about adjacent areas of policy, especially industrial, labor, finance, social services, housing, and education policy. Environmental policy has been the exception that demonstrates the point. Public health agencies initially tested and regulated hazardous substances in workplaces and communities. As a result, state health departments are generally more closely involved with environmental issues than they are with policy for education or social services.

Most state health officials are highly specialized managers rather than major participants in the most important decisions made by the executive branch of government. These are the decisions about what and how much to tax and how to allocate spending among competing claims. In most states, the governor does not regard the senior health official as a trusted political adviser or ally. In many, the health officer does not even hold a cabinet-level position. In hardly any is she or he ever asked by the governor or the legislature to assess the actual or potential impact on health of major policies affecting the economy. Many senior health officials have told me that they do not want such responsibilities. In many states, their colleagues who are responsible for adjacent bureaucratic territory in mental health, developmental disabilities, and treatment for drug and alcohol abuse applaud their technocratic modesty.

The situation appears to be different in the federal government, where a cabinet department is responsible for health. However, federal health officials, other than those with responsibility for the workplace or the environment, have rarely become involved with issues of, for example, economic or industrial policy. Despite the size of the federal health budget, moreover, health policy has rarely been or remained for very long a high priority for a president or his principal staff members (although the Clinton administration may prove to be an exception). The health of the American people has not until recently been regarded, except in speeches, as central to the productivity of the economy or to our ability to compete internationally.

This relative isolation of health policy is the result of a century of giving priority to acute services and according political prominence to groups that provided them. The people who created and maintained health policy for the past century had a vested interest in isolating health politics from other arenas of politics. The people who provided health services used the results of scientific progress to alleviate pain and postpone death. The benefits of health policy seemed, on compelling evidence, to be self-evident and distinctive.

I urge an end to the isolation of health policy. Preventing and managing chronic illness and disability should be regarded as a central purpose of public policy, and therefore of general government, with measurable implications for economic productivity, international competitiveness, and national morale.[24]

The individuals and institutions who provide health care operate public services. Like the consumers of many other public services, people who need health care are often in vulnerable situations; they may lack alternative providers or information on which to make judgments, or they may be under stress. Because health care is a public service, its regulation cannot be entrusted, as it has been for most of the past century, mainly to organizations dominated by people who provide it.[25]

The people who control budgets and appropriations in the executive and legislative branches of government and in the private sector need more timely and precise advice about how their decisions affect the health of particular populations. They may sometimes decide, after public debate, to exchange adverse health effects for economic benefits; but they should know what they are doing. It has not always been unpopular for workers to risk some of their health and safety in order to preserve their jobs. People who drive, fly, eat, worry, and live under stress do that all the time. But how much health do we want to purchase, and with what trade-offs? And what is the best estimate of the cost of alternative policies, and who will pay for them?

There are a few current examples of the new approach to health policy that I am suggesting. In some states, health officers and executives of superagencies, including public health agencies, operate prominently in general government. New York, Maryland, and California have been examples. In several states, governors have taken leadership in health policy. Hawaii, Florida, Minnesota, and Vermont are instances. In a few cities, business leaders and insurers have coalesced with some health sector leaders to reduce costs and improve quality in hospital services. Cleveland and Rochester have such coalitions. A coalition advocating changes in the priorities of health policy has the best chance of success in states with powerful public health agencies and committed governors, senior legislators, and business leaders. The redistribution of resources from hospitals and medical subspecialties to preventing and managing chronic illness may have to proceed state by state, simply because many of the levers for change are in state law and appropriations.[26]

Health policy could, of course, become considerably more responsive to chronic illness and disability without a major change in the priority accorded to it by government and business. For most of the past century, health policy has changed incrementally under the shared leadership of providers and their allies in the private sector and in government. Providers and their allies have made many accommodations to chronic illness and disability. Much more accommodation is possible within the current politics of health affairs. Many hospitals, for example, have been diversifying into long-term and primary care for a decade. Other examples include prominent group and staff model health maintenance organizations, such as Kaiser-Permanente and the Harvard Community Health Plan. These organizations, though not all HMOs, provide a great deal of appropriate care for persons with chronic illness, but remain relatively parsimonious in their use of resources. Similarly, new forms of home and community-based care that emphasize independent (or "interdependent") living are gaining support from large and venerable agencies like the Visiting Nurse Service of New York. A health system that addresses chronic illness more effectively is, optimists could argue, being created within the terms of the health policy compromise of the past generation.

Gradual, voluntary accommodation may, however, address the burden of chronic illness at the price of a vast increase in the cost of health services to our society. We are accommodating the burden now mainly by adding new services and hoping that, in time, the array of unnecessary facilities, technology, and specialists will decrease. Accommodation has, so far, meant creating a more responsive, and often cost-effective, chronic care system alongside the existing acute care system.

More thoroughgoing accommodation to the burden of chronic illness would require explicit changes in what we value. It would require us to share responsibility for each other's needs and aspirations in new ways. Each individual and each of our institutions would have to become more accountable for actions that affect health and the inevitable illness and disability that accompany it. However desirable such change may be, it is unlikely to occur, and certainly not very quickly.

In preceding chapters, I analyzed the history of current health policies and politics. I used the methods and evidence of the social sciences as rigorously as I could. In this chapter, I have advocated changes in policy and politics. I have generalized from both the research literature and my experience in federal and state government, universities, and, recently, philanthropy. The two aspects of my experience, research and public affairs, convince me that Americans should share more responsibility for taking care of each other. Our individual desires and aspirations make it imperative that we act more effectively in our collective interest. I do not advocate either for big government or for small, or for more or less reliance on the public or the private sectors. Rather, I write on behalf of using all of our moral, economic, professional, and institutional resources more wisely in order to postpone suffering and prevent premature death.

Note on Methods and Sources

I tried to make this book credible by grounding it in research. I tried to make it accessible by limiting my use of the conventions of scholarly writing. I could have written a much longer book, adding to the authority of my claims by including more evidence on their behalf. I did research for such a book but chose not to write it. I spent considerable time in archives and research libraries, reading boxes and folders of unpublished sources and many published government documents and articles in medical journals. I had energetic research assistants who found and summarized articles and pamphlets and, occasionally, worked alongside me in archives.

I prefer to select and study archival sources personally, for two reasons. The first is that I enjoy, enormously, handling sources that are handwritten or in typescript or, best of all, a combination of both. Such work gives me the thrill of being vicariously present when history was made. Second, if the equivalent of the smoking guns of criminal law are to be found in research on the history of policy, they will be found only as a result of research in archival sources. The more experienced and attentive the scholar, the more likely it is that he or she will find an astonishing document.

The primary sources I quote or paraphrase are either the rare smoking gun or, more frequently, statements that—because they appear so frequently in the sources—document attitudes and opinions that were important because many people held them. I use endnotes sparingly: to cite documents I have not cited in previous publications or to direct readers to secondary literature, by myself and others, in which they will find citations to relevant primary sources.

Here are more extensive comments on the methods and sources of each chapter.

1. From Consensus to Disarray: A Century of Health Policy

This chapter begins with accounts of imaginary meetings. These meetings are not "counterfactuals" or "thought experiments," however. Every statement I make about each of them is grounded in primary and secondary sources. These imaginary meetings had a real model. On July 21, 1949, everyone who mattered in public and private health affairs in the United States met in New York City to discuss how best to distribute and study the new wonder drug Cortisone. I found the minutes of this meeting in the A. N. Richards Papers at the Archives of the University of Pennsylvania (Box 30). This meeting was the closest I have seen to an assembly of what Marxists have called, usually in metaphor, the "executive committee of the ruling class." I fantasized that similar meetings have occurred but that scholars have not yet found records of them. I explored this fantasy in lectures, asking audiences, "If you had attended a meeting about the priorities of health policy in 1890, where would you have placed your bets? How would you place them now?" Eventually, I constructed the two meetings in this chapter from primary and secondary sources about other contemporary occasions.

Photographs hang in the corridors outside the meetings of 1895 and 1995 because I am convinced that they are revealing primary sources. In *Photographing Medicine: Images and Power in Britain and America since 1840* (Greenwich, Conn.: Greenwood Press, 1988), Christopher Lawrence and I adapted the methods of historians of photographs to the study of medical images. We explained why photographs are not privileged depictions of reality but are instead highly contrived objects (they are, in current jargon, "socially constructed").

I acknowledge some of my debts to secondary sources and to scholars in the text and endnotes of this chapter. Several acknowledgments transcend numbered notes. John Burnham, Gerald Grob, and Rosemary Stevens have for many years contributed to my thinking about the issues that I address in this chapter. Robert H. Ebert and John D. Stoeckle, illustrious physicians, have tried to teach me how to avoid being accused unjustly of criticizing their profession.

2. The Paradox of Health Policy, 1900–1950

The first section of this chapter presents as accessibly as I could the results of research that A. E. Birne and I conducted in 1990. I asked Birne to collect the published data she could find about mortality and morbidity in the United States in the twentieth century. Then we tried to adapt this disparate information so that it could be compared over time. We intend to publish the detailed results of this inquiry, which will be of modest use to specialists.

Next I discuss the National Health Survey of the late 1930s. The survey is a neglected resource for historians. It is not clear what happened to the raw data. I obtained most of my information about the survey from the official papers of its director, George Perrott, who removed them from the Public Health Service upon his retirement and then donated them to the National Library of Medicine on his death.

Data about health policy and public health administration between the 1920s and 1940s are drawn mainly from these sources: Record Groups 90 (U.S. Public Health Service) and 443 (National Institutes of Health), National Archives of the United States, Washington, D.C.; George St. J. Perrott Papers, National Library of Medicine, Bethesda, Maryland; papers of the Committee on the Public Health, New York Academy of Medicine, New York; Milbank Memorial Fund Papers, Sterling Library, Yale University, New Haven, Connecticut; the papers of Margaret Klem, Harvard Medical Archives, Countway Library, Boston; and the corporate archives of Empire Blue Cross and Blue Shield in New York.

Almost all the data about mobilizing a constituency for chronic disabling disease come from unpublished sources, since these activities have not been written about by historians. Important archival sources include the papers of Louis Dublin, Ernest Dalland, and Alan Gregg at the National Library of Medicine; the papers of Alfred E. Cohn, Herbert S. Gasser, the Rockefeller Foundation (including Alan Gregg's official diaries), the Commonwealth Fund, and Sloan Kettering/Memorial Hospital, at the Rockefeller Archives Center, Tarrytown, New York; the papers of Mayor Fiorello H. La Guardia in the New York City Municipal Archives; and the papers of S. S. Goldwater in the archives of Empire Blue Cross, New York.

My collaborator for the research on Cortisone was Marcia Meldrum. We may eventually publish a more extensive version of our work. Major collections of primary sources about Cortisone include the Alfred Newton Richards Papers in the archives of the University of Pennsylvania, Philadelphia; the Walter Bauer Papers in the Countway Library; and the papers of the federal Food and Drug Administration, which are not in the National Archives and can be obtained by consultation with the FDA historian, Suzanne White, in Bethesda.

Mary Grace Kovar and Ronald W. Wilson helped me understand, though still imperfectly, the meaning and limitations of historical statistics about morbidity and mortality. Leon Sokoloff, a distinguished expert on arthritis, helped me understand the scientific issues in the Cortisone debate.

3. The Health Policy Compromise, 1950–1975

Much of this chapter is based on printed primary sources, especially contemporary medical literature, pamphlets, and journalism. The papers of Bess Furman Armstrong at the National Library of Medicine are an unusual combination of printed and unpublished sources. In the 1950s, the U.S. Public Health Service commissioned Armstrong, a former reporter for the *New York Times*, to write its history. Her papers include drafts of her book, unpublished public documents given to her during her research, and her notes of interviews with important contemporaries.

Other pertinent archival sources for this period in the United

States include the papers of Alan Gregg, Rollo Dyer, William Sebrell, the Lasker Awards, the Association of State and Territorial Health Officers, and the American Association of Medical Colleges at the National Library of Medicine; Record Groups 56 (Department of the Treasury), 51 (Bureau of the Budget), 90 (United States Public Health Service), and 443 (National Institutes of Health) at the National Archives of the United States; the Alan Gregg diaries and Rockefeller Foundation papers at the Rockefeller Archives Center, Tarrytown, New York; the papers of Leona Baumgartner at the Harvard Medical Archives, Countway Library, Boston; the papers of Mary E. Switzer at the Schlesinger Library of Radcliffe College, Cambridge, Massachusetts; and the papers of Louis H. Pink and C. Douglas Colman in the archives of Empire Blue Cross and Blue Shield in New York.

Archival sources for policy in the United Kingdom include the papers of the Multiple Sclerosis Society, Sir Thomas Lewis, Sir Edward Mellanby, and George Pickering in the Contemporary Medical Archives Center at the Wellcome Library and Institute for the History of Medicine in London; the papers of the Ministry of Health in the Public Record Office at Kew; and the papers of Trevor Howell and Lord Amulree at the Archives of the British Geriatrics Society in London.

Many people have helped me understand this period. Kenneth Ludmerer and Edward Berkowitz shared their extraordinary knowledge of primary sources on, respectively, the history of medical education and of disability policy. Rosemary Stevens and David Rosner were my partners in planning and conducting a multi-year study of Empire Blue Cross, from which I derive much of what I write about the history of insurance. Edward Werner was both a participant in and a witness to the history of health insurance in these years. Robert H. Ebert has extraordinary knowledge of medical science and education in the third quarter of the century. Irving Zola and David Mechanic helped me understand the changing sociological concept of the sick role. Richard Wolfe of the Countway Library is a rare archivist who accords trusted scholars access to collections of sources that have not yet been processed. Informants in Britain include Michael Ashley-Miller, Raymond Illisley, and, in this as in so many other projects, Rudolf Klein.

4. Health Policy in Disarray, 1975–1993

Because primary sources from these years are not yet accessible in archives, I have relied on conversations, journalism, and personal experience as a participant or close observer of some of the events I describe here.

Many people helped me understand the events I describe here. Kenneth Ludmerer and Robert H. Ebert shared their knowledge of medical education. Eli Ginzberg has special insight into the history of the supply of health services and especially of physicians. Jeremiah Milbank, Jr., and Chris K. Olander have educated me about the values and policy preferences of free-market conservatives. Daniel Schaffer was my collaborator in understanding the links between tax and health policy. Deborah Stone taught me about the concept of being at risk. Many people contributed to my understanding of AIDS; I have special thanks for Ronald Bayer and for my collaborators, Elizabeth Fee and Emily H. Thomas. I have learned about disability policy from David Rothman, Jane West, and Irving Kenneth Zola. Howard Oaks and I talked about the politics of Baby Jane Doe each day during the six months that she was a patient at University Hospital at Stony Brook.

5. Prospects for Policy

This chapter is based entirely on conversations, personal experience, and material in the general and health sector press.

The Milbank Memorial Fund commissioned some of the research I use—for example, by Brian Abel-Smith, Jack A. Meyer, Thomas Ricketts, James Robinson, Louise Russell, Sally Stearns, Mary Stuart, Emily Thomas, and Edward Yelin. My knowledge about acute care that causes harm owes a great deal to the Milbank Memorial Fund's efforts to bring the work of Ian Chalmers and his colleagues on pregnancy and childbirth to the attention of policy makers. Ruth Hanft, Jane Sisk, Barbara Stocking, and

Jonathan Lomas have carried out that work. Similarly, Virginia Beardshaw gave me information about progress in redistributing resources to care for chronic illness in London (described in chapter 3 but important to my thinking about this chapter), as part of a joint project of King Edward's Hospital Fund for London and the Milbank Memorial Fund. Ken Judge of the King's Fund has been vital to that project, as was Robert Maxwell, especially in its initial conceptualization. I know much more about recent state initiatives in health policy as a result of the work of the Milbank Memorial Fund—in particular the research of Howard Leichter and Lawrence D. Brown—and the comments of many of the public officials I name in the next paragraph. Kathleen S. Andersen and Robert A. Fordham of the staff of the Milbank Memorial Fund have been central to this work.

Many conversations have contributed to this chapter. The individuals I credit do not necessarily share my views. Charles Bruner, Lee Greenfield, and David Hollister have, over many years, helped me understand how elected officials like themselves ask and answer the "so what?" question about ideas and information thrust upon them. Rachel Block, Molly Coye, Mark Gibson, Mary Stuart, and Jane West have been eager to discuss how policy is made. Rosemary Stevens has many insights into the limits of contemporary policy. Larry Gostin has fresh ideas about public health law and policy. Similarly, Ann Scitovsky has been my mentor in understanding the costs of illness. I have been routinely enlightened by Carl Schramm, about insurance policy and politics; John Ball and Philip R. Lee, about medical politics and general health policy reform; Fitzhugh Mullan, about physician supply; Steven Schroeder, about primary care and medical specialization; Linda Aiken, about nursing policy and politics and its links to broader issues; Gordon DeFriese and Robert Lawrence, about prevention; and David Rothman, about the recent history of biomedical ethics. Donna I. Regenstreiff helped me understand local initiatives by existing health care organizations to redistribute resources. David Lawrence and Merwyn (Mitch) Greenlick improved my understanding of Kaiser-Permanente, the largest example of the oldest extant form of managed care. Philip H. N.

Wood talked with me at length about his work for the World
Health Organization to make the language of medicine take account of the burden of chronic disabling illness.

I have surely—though inadvertently—left the names of valued
colleagues off this list or one for another chapter. Please accept
my apologies.

Notes

Chapter 1

1. This imaginary meeting is grounded in primary sources and also in an extensive secondary literature that includes the following recent contributions: Daniel M. Fox, *Health Policies, Health Politics: The Experience of Britain and America, 1911–1965* (Princeton, N.J.: Princeton University Press, 1986), and "Medical Institutions and the State," in *Encyclopedia of the History of Medicine*, ed. W. Bynum and R. Porter (London: Routledge, 1993), in press; Kenneth Ludmerer, *Learning to Heal* (New York: Basic Books, 1985); Charles Rosenberg, *The Care of Strangers: The Rise of American Medicine* (New York: Basic Books, 1985); Paul Starr, *The Social Transformation of American Medicine* (New York: Basic Books, 1982); and Rosemary Stevens, *In Sickness and in Wealth: American Hospitals in the Twentieth Century* (New York: Basic Books, 1989). The comments on the significance and interpretation of photographs are extended in Daniel M. Fox and Christopher Lawrence, *Images and Power: Photographing Medicine in Britain and the United States since 1850* (Greenwich, Conn.: Greenwood Press, 1988). I omit the many important articles in journals from this list, mainly because many of these are cited in the above books. A recent article that is not is John Harley Warner, "The Fall and Rise of Professional Mastery: Epistemology, Authority, and the Emergence of Laboratory Medicine in Nineteenth-Century America," in *The Laboratory Revolution in Medicine*, ed. A. Cunningham and P. Williams (Cambridge, England: Cambridge University Press, 1992).

2. What follows is based on both a rich literature and personal experience. Among recent books, Stevens's *In Sickness and in Wealth* is the most pertinent. I have addressed and documented related issues in "AIDS and the American Health Polity: The History and Prospects of a Crisis of Authority," in *AIDS: The Burdens of History*, ed. Elizabeth Fee and Daniel M. Fox (Berkeley: University of California Press, 1988), and "Betting on Our Nation's Health Policy: With and Without Data," in *Proceedings of the 1991 Public Health Conference on Records and Statistics* (Washington, D.C.: U.S. Department of Health and Human Services, National Center for Health Statistics, 1992).

3. Starr, in *The Social Transformation of American Medicine*, summarizes the evidence for physicians' incomes earlier in the century.

4. I have described the close relationship between biomedical research policy and disease in "The Politics of the NIH Extramural Program, 1937–1950," *Journal of the History of Medicine and Allied Sciences* 42 (October 1987): 447–66.

5. For a more extensive discussion of ideology as it bears on research on health policy, see Daniel M. Fox, "Health Policy and the Politics of Research in the United States," *Journal of Health Politics, Policy and Law* 15 (Fall 1990): 481–99.

6. See Fox, "Health Policy and the Politics of Research," for recent literature on using knowledge to inform policy.

7. Stevens, *In Sickness and in Wealth*, p. 357.

8. Fox, *Health Policies, Health Politics*, Introduction.

9. Daniel M. Fox, "Health Policy and Changing Epidemiology in the United States: Chronic Disease in the Twentieth Century," in *Unnatural Causes: The Three Leading Killer Diseases in America*, ed. R. Maulitz (New Brunswick, N.J.: Rutgers University Press, 1989).

10. Sources for these definitions are listed in Daniel M. Fox, "Financing Health Services for the Chronically Ill and Disabled: A History of Political Accommodation," *Milbank Quarterly* 67, supp. 2, part 2 (1989): 257–89.

11. Ann G. Carmichael, "Human Disease in the World outside Asia: European Mortality Decline, 1700–1900," in *The Cam-*

bridge World History of Human Disease, ed. Kenneth F. Kiple (Cambridge: Cambridge University Press, 1993), p. 286.

12. M. S. R. Hutt and D. P. Burkitt, *The Geography of Noninfectious Disease* (Oxford: Oxford University Press, 1986), p. 1.

13. Kiple, *Cambridge World History,* p. 6.

14. Gerald Grob, *From Asylum to Community: Mental Health Policy in Modern America* (Princeton, N.J.: Princeton University Press, 1991).

15. Robert J. Maxwell, review of Fox's *Health Policies, Health Politics, Lancet,* 2, October 10, 1987, p. 828.

16. As I will describe in subsequent chapters, I am merely one among many people who have advocated higher priority for chronic illness. The literature that I have collected on this subject spans a period of almost a century. Advocacy for this position is commonplace at the present time. Specifically, I call attention to the important seminal work of Anselm Strauss in this area. Strauss's articles on the neglect of chronic disease have been appearing for many years. See, for instance, "Health Policy and Chronic Illness," *Society* 25 (November/December 1987): 33–39.

Chapter 2

1. I have chosen a parsimonious citation strategy for this book. The purpose of the strategy is to inform expert readers without cluttering the text with numbers. Thus, I cite quotations or extensive paraphrases from primary sources only when I have not previously cited them in one of the articles I published during the years I explored the information and ideas that I synthesize in this book. When I have previously cited a source, the endnote refers readers to the published article in which that source was cited. Similarly, I do not cite secondary sources for information that is generally accepted by people who do research on health policy and its history. But I cite secondary sources that offer new insights, or are controversial, or are, at this writing, unpublished.

The quotation in this paragraph is from "The Need of Hospital Provision for Chronic Patients," Report of the Public Health, Hospital and Budget Committee of the New York Academy of Medicine to the Commissioner of Health of New York City (New York Academy of Medicine Archives, CPH CD 191430), April 1914.

2. *Vital Statistics in the United States, 1940–1960* (Washington, D.C.: Department of Health, Education and Welfare, National Center for Health Statistics, 1968), p. 79.

3. Ibid.

4. Ibid.

5. Anne-Emanuelle Birne and Daniel M. Fox, "Chronic Disease Morbidity and Mortality in the United States since 1900," unpublished paper, 1991. This paper is the source of the data in the following paragraphs, except where other sources are cited. We hope eventually to publish the documentation for this paper.

6. James C. Riley, *Sickness, Recovery and Death: A History and Forecast of Ill Health* (Iowa City: University of Iowa Press, 1989). For the current controversy about how to interpret morbidity data, see S. Ryan Johansson, "The Health Transition: The Cultural Inflation of Morbidity during the Decline of Mortality," *Health Transition Review* 1, no. 1 (1991): 39–68; and James C. Riley's reply, "From a High Mortality Regime to a High Morbidity Regime: Is Culture Everything in Sickness," *Health Transition Review* 2, no. 2 (1992): 71–89.

7. The most convenient of several sources for the data on the National Health Survey in this and the following paragraphs is *The National Health Survey, 1935–36: The Magnitude of the Chronic Disease Problem in the United States*, preliminary reports, Sickness and Medical Care Series, Bulletin no. 6 (Washington, D.C.: Division of Public Health Methods, National Institutes of Health, U.S. Public Health Service, 1938), pp. 1–19.

8. Quotations cited in Daniel M. Fox, "Financing Health Services for the Chronically Ill and Disabled: A History of Political Accommodation," *Milbank Quarterly* 67, supp. 2, part 2 (1989): 257–89.

9. See Ronald W. Wilson and Thomas F. Drury, "Interpreting Trends in Illness and Disability: Health Statistics and Health Status," *Annual Review of Public Health* 5 (1984): 83–106. See also Dorothy P. Rice and Mitchell P. LaPlante, "Chronic Illness, Disability and Increasing Longevity," in *The Economics and Ethics*

of Long-Term Care and Disability, ed. Sean Sullivan and Marion Ein Lewin (Washington, D.C.: American Enterprise Institute, 1988). An important unpublished study is Richard W. Osborn, "A Time Series Analysis of Population Morbidity and Disability," Department of Preventive Medicine and Biostatistics, Faculty of Medicine, University of Toronto, 1991. Osborn finds that "in direct opposition to the popular model we find there to be an *increasing* prevalence of chronic conditions over the time period [1969–81]" (p. 18).

10. See Daniel M. Fox, *Health Policies, Health Politics: The Experience of Britain and America, 1911–1965* (Princeton, N.J.: Princeton University Press, 1986), and "Medical Institutions and the State," in *Encyclopedia of the History of Medicine,* ed. W. Bynum and R. Porter (London: Routledge, 1993); Kenneth Ludmerer, *Learning to Health* (New York: Basic Books, 1985); Charles Rosenberg, *The Care of Strangers: The Rise of American Medicine* (New York: Basic Books, 1985); Paul Starr, *The Social Transformation of American Medicine* (New York: Basic Books, 1982); and Rosemary Stevens, *In Sickness and in Wealth: American Hospitals in the Twentieth Century* (New York: Basic Books, 1989).

11. There is an extensive literature health reform in this period. See especially the works by Stevens, Starr, and Fox cited in the preceding note. For what follows on early health insurance, the literature is sparse. See, however, D. M. Fox, David Rosner, and R. A. Stevens, "Between Public and Private: A Half Century of Blue Cross and Blue Shield in New York: Introduction," *Journal of Health Politics, Policy and Law* 16 (Winter 1991): 643–50, and the other papers assembled in the same issue of this journal.

12. The source for Parran's astonishing quote is the transcript of a radio broadcast he made on the Columbia network, July 19, 1938, in Box 169, NIH Government File, Record Group 443, National Archives of the United States.

13. The quotes in the next several paragraphs are cited in Fox, "Financing Health Services."

14. For citations to most of the quotations and paraphrases in this section, see D. M. Fox, "Health Policy and Changing Epide-

miology in the United States: Chronic Disease in the Twentieth Century," in *Unnatural Causes: The Three Leading Killer Diseases in America*, ed. R. Maulitz (New Brunswick, N.J.: Rutgers University Press, 1989), and "Financing Health Services." The story I tell in this section is, however, based mainly on extensive reading in archival sources. For a list of these sources, see the Note on Methods and Sources at the end of this book.

15. A. E. Cohn, Memorandum for a meeting with Robert Maynard Hutchins, May 1935, Cohn Papers, Box 18 (7), Rockefeller Archives Center, Tarrytown, N.Y.

16. Ernst P. Boas, *Treatment of the Patient Past Fifty* (Chicago: Year Book Publishers, 1941), p. 5.

17. For citations see Daniel M. Fox, "The Politics of the NIH Extramural Program, 1937–1950," *Journal of the History of Medicine and Allied Sciences* 42 (October 1987): 447–66.

18. As I described in "The Politics of the NIH Extramural Program," the participants in these events subsequently remembered them as less controversial than the evidence in manuscript sources reveals, and as more focused on science than on chronic disease. A telling confirmation of my point, however, is in the "closing comment" in James A. Shannon's memoir of the 1950s, "The National Institutes of Health: Some Critical Years, 1955–57," *Science* 237 (August 21, 1987): 865–68. Shannon takes for granted the centrality of chronic disease to NIH policy: "Within the complexities of the many chronic diseases of concern to NIH . . . the immediate objectives were to increase the order of magnitude of the [research] effort, provide a broader base of understanding of the biological systems involved, and, with an increasing knowledge of the natural history of disease, approach its [chronic disease's] solution in an opportunistic fashion."

19. Primary sources about lobbying on behalf of NIH are in the Mary Switzer Papers, Schlesinger Library, Radcliffe College. For mental health policy in these years, see Gerald Grob, *From Asylum to Community: Mental Health Policy in Modern America* (Princeton, N.J.: Princeton University Press, 1991).

20. Daniel M. Fox, "Sharing Governmental Authority: Blue Cross and Hospital Planning in New York City," *Journal of Health Politics, Policy and Law* 16 (Winter 1991): 719–46.

21. For documentation on support for these priorities, see Fox, *Health Policies, Health Politics*, chaps. 7 and 9.

22. David Seegal and Arthur R. Wertheim, "Prospects for the Prevention of Chronic Disease," paper presented at the conference on Preventive Aspects of Chronic Disease, sponsored by the Commission on Chronic Illness, the National Health Council, and the U.S. Public Health Service, Chicago, March 12–14, 1951.

23. Daniel M. Fox and Marcia Meldrum, "Cortisone 1949–1950: History and the Politics of Medical Progress," paper presented at the annual meeting of the American Association for the History of Medicine, Baltimore, May 1990. In conversation, Kenneth Ludmerer noted that the Mayo Clinic, unlike Merck, surrendered its patent claims to Cortisone in the public interest. Physicians' ethical views of their public obligation changed markedly, he continued, between 1947 and the events I discuss in chapter 4.

Chapter 3

1. For citations not otherwise noted, see Daniel M. Fox, "Financing Health Services for the Chronically Ill and Disabled: A History of Political Accommodation," *Milbank Quarterly* 67, supp. 2, part 2 (1989): 257–89, and "Health Policy and Changing Epidemiology in the United States: Chronic Disease in the Twentieth Century," in *Unnatural Causes: The Three Leading Killer Diseases in America*, ed. R. Maulitz (New Brunswick, N.J.: Rutgers University Press, 1989). For a general history of these issues, see Fox, *Health Policies, Health Politics: The Experience of Britain and America, 1911–1965* (Princeton, N.J.: Princeton University Press, 1986); and Rosemary Stevens, *In Sickness and in Wealth: American Hospitals in the Twentieth Century* (New York: Basic Books, 1989).

2. Kenneth Ludmerer, "American Medical Education in the Twentieth Century: A Prospectus," unpublished manuscript, 1992, p. 9.

3. For citations on rehabilitation and disability in this period, see Edward Berkowitz and Daniel M. Fox, "The Politics of Social

Security Expansion: Social Security Disability Insurance, 1935–1986," *Journal of Policy History* 14 (Summer 1989): 239–60.

4. *The Multiple Screening Idea* (New York: Health Information Foundation, n.d. but probably 1952), copy in the Douglas Colman Papers, Empire Blue Cross/Blue Shield Archives.

5. Eli Ginzberg, *A Pattern for Hospital Care: Final Report of the New York State Hospital Study* (New York: Columbia University Press, 1949), p. 180.

6. The sources quoted in this and the next two paragraphs are in Leona Baumgartner Papers, Organization File to 1962, file labeled "Interdepartmental Health Council," Harvard Medical Archives, Countway Library, Boston.

7. Talcott Parsons, *The Social System* (New York: Free Press, 1951), chap. 10. This reading of Parsons places him in the context of his time as a social scientist. It contradicts the more frequent reading of Parsons as a normative lawgiver. This is not the place to defend at any length the benefits of using the methods of intellectual history to analyze the social science of an earlier generation. But such a defense would note that Parsons was indebted to Henry Sigerist's classic paper of 1929, "The Special Position of the Sick" (in *Henry E. Sigerist on the Sociology of Medicine*, ed. M. I. Roemer [New York: MD Publications, 1960]). Sigerist, writing in an earlier generation than Parsons, emphasized that the "goal of medical intervention is the restoration of function." Parsons, observing several decades of popular assimilation of optimistic ideas about medical progress, replaced the concept of function with the much more demanding task of "getting well."

8. Parsons, *The Social System*, p. 431, n. 7.

9. See pertinent papers in Irving K. Zola, *Socio-Medical Inquiries: Reflections, Recollections and Reconsiderations* (Philadelphia: Temple University Press, 1983).

10. W. C. Arntz to Elmer B. Staats, February 5, 1960, Record Group 51, Bureau of the Budget Series 51.3a, Box 19, National Archives of the United States.

11. David Bell to John F. Kennedy, March 10, 1961, Record Group 51, Bureau of the Budget Series 61.1a, R5-2/2, Box 45, National Archives.

12. Internal White House correspondence reveals that opposition to crash programs remained strong but ineffective. William Cannon, an official in the Bureau of the Budget, insisted that the activities on behalf of diffusing technology for these diseases "would accomplish little and would actively harm our efforts to keep the NIH budget under executive branch control." Cannon believed that the "problems posed by cancer, heart disease and stroke are primarily research problems" for which NIH already had enough money (William Cannon to Myer Feldman, September 30 and July 26, 1963, Record Group 51, Bureau of the Budget Series 69.1, Box 82, National Archives). For an analogous view, expressed on behalf of community mental health programs as a solution to the problems of the severely mentally ill, see Gerald Grob, *From Asylum to Community: Mental Health Policy in Modern America* (Princeton, N.J.: Princeton University Press, 1991).

13. Again, this account is based on manuscript sources in the National Archives, which I cite in telling the larger story in "International Perspectives," in *Human Resources for Health: Defining the Future*, ed. C. M. Evarts et al. (Washington, D.C.: Association of Academic Health Centers, 1992).

14. D. M. Fox, "Sharing Governmental Authority: Blue Cross and Hospital Planning in New York City," *Journal of Health Politics, Policy and Law* 16 (Winter 1991): 719–46.

15. The evaluators were Arthur D. Little, Inc., and a nonprofit firm called the Organization for Social and Technical Innovation. I was a principal in the latter and principal investigator of the sole-source contract to evaluate CHP. Everything reported in this paragraph is personal observation.

16. Fox, "Financing Health Services." I am indebted to James Maxwell's still unpublished history of Blue Cross in New York for some of what follows. Much of what I say about the Blues and the commercials is a result of documents in the archives at Empire Blue Cross and Blue Shield, notably the papers of Louis Pink and Douglas Colman.

17. Chester J. Pack, Jr., and Elmo Richardson, *The Presidency of Dwight D. Eisenhower* (Lawrence: University of Kansas Press,

1991), p. 56. See also Gary W. Reichard, *Politics as Usual: The Age of Truman and Eisenhower* (Arlington Heights, Ill.: Harlan Davidson, 1988), pp. 86–87.

18. Stephen Ambrose, *Eisenhower: The President*, vol. 3 (New York: Simon and Schuster, 1984), p. 199.

19. For primary sources on the history of Social Security Disability Insurance, see Berkowitz and Fox, "The Policies of Social Security Expansion."

20. For the literature on Medicare and chronic disease, see Fox, "Financing Health Services." The most recent assessment of this issue is Lawrence R. Jacobs, *A Social Interpretation of Institutional Change: Public Opinion and Policy Making in the Enactment of the British National Health Service Act of 1946 and the American Medicare Act of 1965.* Ph.D. dissertation, Columbia University, 1990; forthcoming as a book from Cornell University Press.

21. John Francis to William Carey, "Events Leading to the Establishment of the Gottschalk Committee," memorandum, March 18, 1968, Record Group 51, BoB file 60.3a, Box 23, National Archives of the United States.

22. John Francis to Pierre Palmer, August 10, 1967, Record Group 51, BoB file 60.3a, Box 23, National Archives; Richard A. Rettig, "Origins of the Medicare Kidney Disease Entitlement: The Social Security Amendments of 1972," in *Biomedical Politics*, ed. K. E. Hanna (Washington, D.C.: National Academy Press, 1991), 189–90.

23. Sandra Tannenbaum, "Medicaid and Disability: The Unlikely Entitlement," *Milbank Quarterly* 67, supp. 2, part 2 (1989): 288–310.

24. The leading explanations of our health financing policy are assessed, rather differently, in Fox, *Health Policies, Health Politics;* Starr, *Social Transformation of American Medicine;* and several thoughtful works by Hollingsworth, most recently J. Rogers Hollingsworth, Jerald Hage, and Robert A. Hanneman, *State Intervention in Medical Care: Consequences for Britain, France, Sweden, and the United States, 1890–1970* (Ithaca, N.Y.: Cornell University Press, 1990).

25. This section is based mainly on research in the Contemporary Medical History Archives of the Wellcome Institute for the History of Medicine, the British Public Records Office, the archives of the British Geriatric Society, and printed public primary sources in the British Library. I have told the story in more detail in "The Perception of Chronic Illness in Health Policy: Britain and America, 1930s–1960s," in *Program, Papers and Abstracts for the Joint Conference of the British Society for the History of Science and the History of Science Society* (Manchester: BHSS and HSS, 1988).

26. *Report of the Ministry of Health for the Year Ended 1945 Including the Report of the Chief Medical Officer of Health on the State of the Public Health for the Year Ended 1945* (London: Her Majesty's Stationery Office, 1946), pp. 77–78, 81, 13.

27. Interview, Bath, United Kingdom, July 1988.

28. In particular see the papers of Sir Thomas Lewis and Sir Edward Mellanby, both in the Contemporary Medical Archives Center, Wellcome Library and Institute for the History of Medicine, London.

29. Rudolf Klein, *The Politics of the National Health Service*, 2nd ed. (London: Longmans, 1989). I have a special debt to Professor Klein as a result of many conversations with him about health policy in the United States and the United Kingdom.

30. A notable publication that discusses the "young chronic sick" is *Separation of Younger from Older Patients in Hospitals* (London: Her Majesty's Stationery Office, 1975).

31. King's Fund Commission on the Future of London's Acute Health Services, *London Health Care 2010: Changing the Future of Services in the Capital* (London: King Edward's Hospital Fund for London, 1992). An official commission soon recommended that the government accept most of the recommendations by the King's Fund Commission. See Sir Bernard Tominson et al., *Report of the Inquiry into London's Health Service, Medical Education and Research* (London: Her Majesty's Stationery Office, 1992).

32. I am grateful to Dr. Michael Ashley-Miller, secretary of the Nuffield Provincial Hospitals Trust, for conversations that bear on this paragraph.

Chapter 4

1. Advocates of prevention policy frequently get upset when they are confronted with evidence that prevention does not always save money or that rational political actors must consider *when* and in *whose budget* savings occur. For this debate see, for example, Louise Russell, *Educated Guesses* (Berkeley and New York: University of California Press and Milbank Memorial Fund, forthcoming).

2. Theodore R. Marmor, Jerry L. Mashaw, and Philip Harvey, *America's Misunderstood Welfare State* (New York: Basic Books, 1991).

3. Robert Griffith, "Dwight D. Eisenhower and the Corporate Commonwealth," *American Historical Review* 87 (February 1982): 87–122.

4. Walter Dean Burnham, "Into the 1980s with Ronald Reagan," in *The Current Crisis in American Politics* (New York: Oxford University Press, 1982, pp. 273–76), takes a slightly different view of the political history of centralization. He argues that a "momentous transition . . . toward [a] much more active and intrusive federal role in the maintenance of . . . social harmony" took place after 1965. I believe that, for ideological purposes, it began considerably earlier. On Wilbur Cohen, see the forthcoming biography by Edward Berkowitz.

5. On the history of conservative political thought, see George N. Nash, *The Conservative Intellectual Movement in America* (New York: Basic Books, 1976); and Davis W. Reinhard, *The Republican Right since 1945* (Lexington: University Press of Kentucky, 1983). Burnham ("Into the 1980s with Ronald Reagan," p. 280) writes of the "continuing vitality of the American liberal-capitalist political tradition, and the enduring hostility to the state, to organized labor, to the poor that arises from this kind of uncontested cultural hegemony." An important review article on the history of conservative politics is Michael Kazin, "The Grass-Roots Right: New Histories of U.S. Conservatism in the Twentieth Century," *American Historical Review* 97 (February 1992): 136–55.

6. D. M. Fox, *Economists and Health Care* (New York: Prodist, 1979), and "Health Policy and the Politics of Research in the United States," *Journal of Health Politics, Policy and Law* 15 (Fall 1990): 481–99.

7. John C. Burnham, "American Medicine's Golden Age: What Happened to It?" *Science* 215 (March 1982): 1475–77.

8. See Fox, *Health Policies, Health Politics*, chaps. 5 and 7.

9. Similarly, in September 1992, the American College of Physicians, the largest organization of specialists, announced a comprehensive plan for health policy reform, including cost controls, that was immediately dismissed by the White House.

10. For details about alleged profit seeking among physicians, see Bradford H. Gray, *The Profit Motive and Patient Care: The Changing Accountability of Doctors and Hospitals* (Cambridge, Mass.: Harvard University Press, 1991); and Walt Bogdanich, *The Great White Lie: How America's Hospitals Betray Our Trust and Endanger Our Lives* (New York: Simon and Schuster, 1991).

11. D. M. Fox and D. C. Schaffer, "Health Policy and ERISA: Interest Groups and Semi-preemption," *Journal of Health Politics, Policy and Law* 14 (Summer 1989): 239–60.

12. D. M. Fox and D. C. Schaffer, "Tax Policy as Social Policy: Cafeteria Plans, 1987–1985," *Journal of Health Politics, Policy and Law* 12 (Winter 1987): 447–66.

13. For the earlier history of physician self-control of conflicts of interest, see Katherine Ann Durso, "Profit Status in the Early History of Health Maintenance Organizations," Ph.D. diss., Yale University, 1992.

14. K. Ludmerer, "American Medical Education in the Twentieth Century: A Prospectus," unpublished manuscript, 1992, p. 16.

15. Stephen M. Shortell, "Revisiting the Garden: Medicine and Management in the 1990s," *Frontiers of Health Services Management* 7 (Fall 1990): 5.

16. Bogdanich, *The Great White Lie*, p. 136.

17. Jean M. Mitchell and Elton Scott, "New Evidence of the Prevalence and Scope of Physician Joint Ventures," *Journal of the American Medical Association* 268 (July 1, 1992): 80–84.

18. Daniel M. Fox, "Medical Institutions and the State," in *Encyclopedia of the History of Medicine,* ed. W. Bynum and R. Porter (London: Routledge, 1993).

19. Arnold S. Relman, "Self-Referral—What's at Stake?" *New England Journal of Medicine* 327 (November 19, 1992): 1522–24. Relman has written many other articles on this subject.

20. Quoted in Bogdanich, *The Great White Lie,* p. 104, from *Internist,* January 1987, p. 26. Similarly, the General Accounting Office reported in 1992 that "unscrupulous health care providers, including practitioners and medical equipment suppliers, . . . cheat health insurance companies and programs out of billions of dollars annually." See U.S. General Accounting Office, *Health Insurance: Vulnerable Payers Lose Billions to Fraud and Abuse,* Report to the Chairman, Subcommittee on Human Resources and Intergovernmental Relations, Committee on Government Operations, House of Representatives, B-246412 (Washington, D.C.: General Accounting Office, May 7, 1992).

21. Marc Rodwin, *Medicine, Money and Morals: Physicians' Conflict of Interest in the United States* (New York: Oxford University Press, 1993). Instances in point appear regularly in the medical press. For example, "utilization, charges per patient, and profits are higher when physical therapy and rehabilitation facilities are owned by referring physicians": Jean M. Mitchell and Elton Scott, "Physician Ownership of Physical Therapy Services," *Journal of the American Medical Association* 268 (October 21, 1992): 2055–59.

22. Robert Petersdorff, quoted in Daniel M. Fox, "Physicians' Antagonism to Lawyers: AIDS as Irritant and Opportunity," in *AIDS and the Law,* ed. Scott Burris (New Haven, Conn.: Yale University Press, 1987; rev. ed., 1992).

23. I witnessed this event (the lobbyist complaining to the committee about physicians' behavior toward legislators) by accident, because I was attending the executive committee's meeting to address another issue.

24. An extensive correspondence on this subject—including letters by Rockefeller, Gregg, and distinguished scientists—took place between April and August 1948 and is filed in the papers of

the Rockefeller Foundation, R62 200 412 2779, Rockefeller Archives Center, Tarrytown, N.Y.

25. James F. Fries, "The Compression of Morbidity: Near or Far?" *Milbank Quarterly* 67 (Spring 1989): 208–31.

26. Office of Technology Assessment, U.S. Congress, *Impact of Randomized Clinical Trials on Health Policy and Medical Practice: Background Paper*, OTA-BP-H-22 (Washington, D.C.: U.S. Government Printing Office, 1983).

27. See Anne-Emanuelle Birne and Daniel M. Fox, "Chronic Disease Morbidity and Mortality in the United States since 1900," unpublished paper, 1991.

28. World Health Organization, Preamble, *Constitution of the WHO* (Geneva: World Health Organization, 1946).

29. This paragraph and those that follow on this subject owe a great deal to Deborah A. Stone, "At Risk in the Welfare State," *Social Research* 56 (Autumn 1989): 591–633.

30. Similar implications of the increasing prevalence of disability are discussed in a provocative article by Gareth H. Williams, "Disablement and the Ideological Crisis in Health Care," *Social Science and Medicine* 32, no. 4 (1991): 517–24.

31. Daniel M. Fox, "AIDS and the American Health Polity: The History and Prospects of a Crisis of Authority," in *AIDS: The Burdens of History*, ed. E. Fee and D. M. Fox (Berkeley: University of California Press, 1988), and "Chronic Disease and Disadvantage: The New Politics of HIV Infection," *Journal of Health Politics, Policy and Law* 16 (Summer 1990): 341–55.

32. Elizabeth Fee and Daniel M. Fox, "The Contemporary Historiography of AIDS," *Journal of Social History* 23 (Winter 1989): 303–14; D. M. Fox, R. Klein, and P. Day, "The Power of Professionalism: Policies for AIDS in Britain, Sweden and the United States," *Daedalus* 118 (Spring 1989): 93–112.

33. David J. Rothman and Harold Edgar, "Scientific Rigor and Medical Realities: Placebo Trials in Cancer and AIDS Research," in *AIDS: The Making of a Chronic Disease*, ed. E. Fee and D. M. Fox (Berkeley: University of California Press, 1992).

34. Daniel M. Fox, "Health Policy and the New Disability Policy: The Potential for Convergence," in *Social Insurance for the*

Nineties, Proceedings of the Third Conference of the National Academy of Social Insurance (Washington, D.C.: National Academy of Social Insurance, 1992).

35. Daniel M. Fox, ed., "The Baby Jane Doe Papers," *Journal of Health Politics, Policy and Law* 11 (Summer 1986): entire issue. I was a participant in some of the politics of the Baby Jane Doe case as a senior official of the Health Sciences Center of the State University of New York at Stony Brook. David J. Rothman discusses the convergence of disability and health policy around neonatal issues in *Strangers at the Bedside* (New York: Basic Books, 1991), chap. 10.

36. Jane West, ed., *The Americans with Disabilities Act: From Policy to Practice* (New York: Milbank Memorial Fund, 1991).

37. Jane West, *Moving toward the Mainstream: Disability Rights Policy and Politics in the 100th Congress,* final report of a 1989–90 Mary E. Switzer Rehabilitation Research Distinguished Fellowship Grant (Washington, D.C.: U.S. Department of Education, 1992).

Chapter 5

1. John W. Kingdon, *Congressmen's Voting Decisions,* 3rd ed. (Ann Arbor: University of Michigan Press, 1989). Kingdon writes, for example, "The members' own policy attitudes, their own conception of good public policy remained central driving forces in their decisions [p. xi]. . . . Interest groups are important, but mostly when they can claim a constituency connection [p. xiii]. . . . [Legislators] take cues from fellow congressmen . . . and look for consensus in the fields of force that affect them" (p. xiii). See also Carol H. Weiss, ed., *Organizations for Policy Analysis: Helping Government Think* (Newbury Park, Calif.: Sage, 1992), pp. 13–14: "What actually happens depends on the mix of interests, ideologies and institutional procedures in the public domain and on the political will to make things happen."

2. For attitudes toward hospital governance, see Rosemary Stevens, *In Sickness and in Wealth: American Hospitals in the Twentieth Century* (New York: Basic Books, 1989), and "Can the

Government Govern? Lessons from the Formation of the Veterans Administration," *Journal of Health Politics, Policy and Law* 16 (Summer 1991): 281–306.

3. Thomas Ricketts, "The Future of the Small Rural Hospital," unpublished report for the Milbank Memorial Fund, 1992.

4. Mary Stuart, "Redefining Boundaries in the Financing and Care of Diabetes: The Maryland Experience," paper commissioned by the Milbank Memorial Fund, 1992 (under review for publication).

5. Roger A. Rosenblatt, "Specialists or Generalists: On Whom Should We Base the American Health Care System?" *Journal of the American Medical Association* 267 (March 25, 1992): 1665–66. This editorial commented on the findings reported in the same issue (pp. 1624–30) by Sheldon Greenfield et al., "Variations in Resource Utilization among Medical Specialties and Systems of Care."

6. The quote is from Thomas B. Graboys et al., "Results of a Second-Opinion Trial among Patients Recommended for Coronary Angiography," *Journal of the American Medical Association* 268 (November 11, 1992): 2537–40.

7. The most dramatic and well publicized of these studies is the meta-analysis of pregnancy and childbirth directed by Ian Chalmers and his colleagues, based in the newly named Cochrane Center at Oxford University. For a list of interventions that cause harm, see Ian Chalmers, Murray Enkin, and D. Keirse, *Effective Care in Pregnancy and Childbirth*, vol. 2, Appendix 1 (Oxford: Oxford University Press, 1990).

8. Ann Scitovsky, "Medical Care in the Last Twelve Months of Life: The Relation between Age, Functional Status and Medical Care Expenditures," *Milbank Quarterly* 66 (1988): 656; Sally C. Stearns et al., "Hospital Use during the Last Year of Life: Does Implicit Rationing Occur for the Elderly with Poor Prognosis?" report prepared for the Milbank Memorial Fund, 1992 (under review for publication), 21. For anecdotal data about physician, family, and patient complicity in limiting care for patients with poor prognoses, see Robert Zussman, *Intensive Care: Medical Ethics and the Medical Profession* (Chicago: University of Chi-

cago Press, 1992). Zussman argues that care for the terminally ill is in fact negotiated rather than rationed.

9. D. M. Fox and D. C. Schaffer, "Health Policy and ERISA: Interest Groups and Semi-preemption," *Journal of Health Politics, Policy and Law* 14 (Summer 1989): 239–60.

10. Lawrence Jacobs, *A Social Interpretation of Institutional Change* (ch. 3, n. 20).

11. Stephen L. Percy, *Disability, Civil Rights and Public Policy: The Politics of Implementation* (Tuscaloosa: University of Alabama Press, 1989), p. 221.

12. A very persuasive argument that these results are possible without massive institutional, and therefore political, change has been made by Patricia M. Danzon, "Hidden Overhead Costs: Is Canada's System Really Less Expensive?" *Health Affairs* 11 (Spring 1992): 30. Danzon writes: "The . . . common argument that monopoly insurers have lower costs of risk and other functions because of the larger risk pool is inconsistent with the evidence. . . . The survival of both small and large insurers indicates that scale economies from risk pooling are eliminated at fairly small scale or can be achieved through reinsurance."

13. Jack A. Meyer, Sharon Silow-Carroll, and Brian Garrett, *Setting New Priorities in Health Care* (New York: Milbank Memorial Fund, 1993).

14. In an important article, two Canadian economists make this argument (that health care expenditures are less advantageous to the economy than other expenditures are) and add that spending to expand the health sector may itself have negative effects on both the creation of wealth and the health of populations. See Robert G. Evans and Gregory L. Stoddart, "Producing Health, Consuming Health Care," *Social Science and Medicine* 31, no. 12 (1990): 1347–63. A century ago, there seemed to be evidence that spending for health services was good for the general economy. The campaign to eradicate hookworm in the South surely added to the productivity of the work force. The contemporary evidence is less compelling. Disability rights advocates contend that services that permit people to work prevent individual and social costs of dependency. On the other hand, as the popula-

tion ages, a great deal is spent on services to people who are not in the productive economy.

15. Emily H. Thomas and Arlene H. Nolan, "What Is a Hospital? A Profile of Hospitals in the United States," unpublished report to the Milbank Memorial Fund, May 1992. Their calculation of the cost of staffed but empty beds was disputed by other experts. People who treasure futilitarian arguments (the woodwork effect, described in the text, is another) enjoy arguing that changes in policy will have little or no effect. For a stimulating analysis of the reasons these arguments are persuasive, see Albert O. Hirschman, *The Rhetoric of Reaction: Perversity, Futility, Jeopardy* (Cambridge, Mass.: Belknap Press of Harvard University Press, 1991).

Futilitarianism aside, people who have managed or regulated hospitals know that their expenditures per bed, occupied or empty, can be reduced by pressure from payers and regulators who act in the interests of payers. Moreover, such reductions can be made—up to a point that has hardly ever been reached in modern America—without any direct effect on the intensity or even the quality of these services.

16. I am grateful for this observation, and many others in point, to David C. Hollister of the Michigan House of Representatives.

17. World Health Organization, *International Classification of Impairments, Disabilities and Handicaps*, rev. ed. (Geneva: World Health Organization, 1980).

18. Philip H. N. Wood, then at the medical school of the University of Manchester, England, the principal author of the classification, spent considerable time explaining its significance to me in July 1988. Wood and others have published extensively on this subject in the international literature. The significance of the *International Classification of Impairment, Disabilities, and Handicaps* (ICIDH) has been underrated in the United States because it has become the subject of a technical dispute among statisticians. The dispute has precluded it from being used, as it is in many places abroad, as an instrument of administration that implements a new conception of health policy priorities. Anyone

wanting to be informed about the use of the ICIDH in policy making throughout the world should get on the mailing list of the World Health Organization Collaborating Center for the ICIDH, National Council for Public Health, P.O. Box 7100, 2701 AC Zoetermeer, Netherlands. As of September 1992, the center had identified 1,068 articles bearing on the use of the ICIDH for policy in the world medical literature.

19. I am grateful to Charles Fox (no relation), then managing editor of *Road and Track*, for this information in a conversation in 1986. I made a blunder in my telephone conversation with him, asking him to send me a reprint of the article. "A what?" he replied.

20. Both the evidence and the reasons for not exaggerating it are synthesized in Edward Yelin, *Work Disability* (New Brunswick, N.J.: Rutgers University Press, 1992).

21. Data showing the relationship between reductions in the supply of acute care services and reductions in total health care costs are assembled in Brian Abel-Smith, "Cost Containment and New Priorities in the European Community," *Milbank Quarterly* 70, no. 3 (1992): 393–416. See also United States General Accounting Office, *Health Care Spending Control: The Experience of France, Germany and Japan*, GAO/HRD-92-9 (Washington, D.C.: General Accounting Office, 1991).

22. For a history of and remedies for the problem of an oversupply of specialists, see Eli Ginzberg, "Physician Supply Policies and Health Reform," *Journal of the American Medical Association* 268 (December 2, 1992): 3115–18.

23. In 1971, government officials in London demonstrated the role of political will in forming such a coalition when they mobilized support for changing priorities in acute services. I describe and cite sources for the London coalition at the end of chapter 3. A promising nationwide alliance of philanthropists and health care providers in the United States is the National Chronic Care Consortium, based in Bloomington, Minnesota. It remains to be seen, however, whether the large hospitals that comprise most of the institutional members of this consortium are more interested in institutional maintenance or in genuine redistribution of resources.

24. There is some evidence that an emphasis on preventing and managing chronic illness would have beneficial effects. The Centers for Disease Control and Prevention in the U.S. Department of Health and Human Services estimates that "eliminating a single risk factor for each of nine key chronic diseases could reduce mortality from these causes by 47%, from 427 per 100,000 persons to 224 per 100,000." Editorial, "Chronic Disease Prevention and Control Activities—United States, 1989," *Morbidity and Mortality Weekly Report* 40 (October 18, 1991): 697–700.

25. I am grateful to James C. Robinson for new ideas about uncertainty and how to make better policy to address it. His papers on this subject include "A New Institutional Economics Health Care," 1992.

26. Harry Nelson et al., *The States That Could Not Wait: Health Reform in Hawaii, Oregon, Minnesota, Vermont, and Florida* (New York: Milbank Memorial Fund, 1993).

Index

Compositor:	ComCom, Inc.
Text:	10/13 Aster
Display:	Helvetica Condensed and Aster
Printer:	Haddon Craftsmen, Inc.
Binder:	Haddon Craftsmen, Inc.